FITNESS AND TRAINING

MIND AND BODY FITNESS

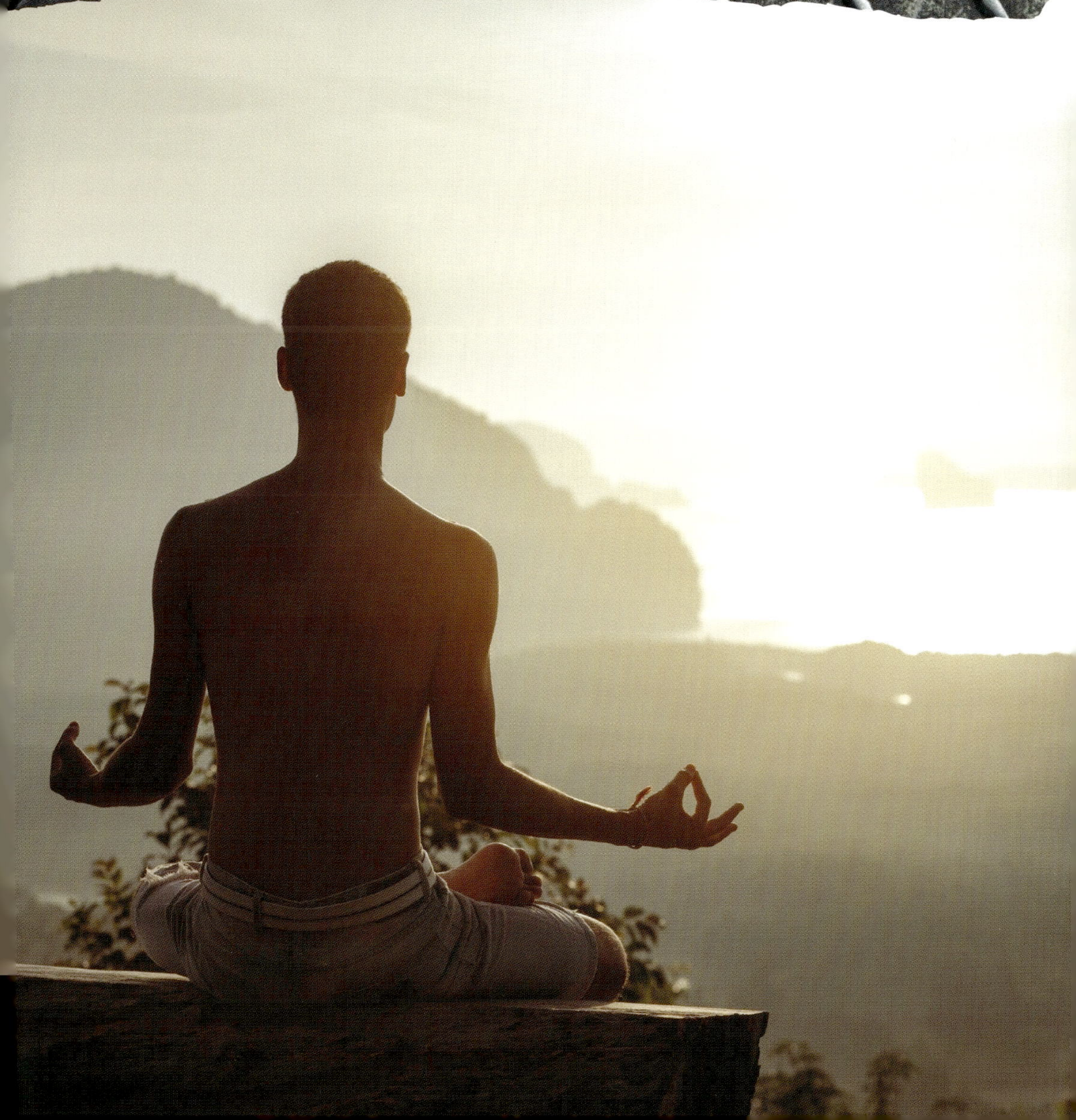

FITNESS AND TRAINING

Core Training
Endurance Training
Fitness and Nutrition
High-Energy Workouts
High-Intensity Interval Training (HIIT)
Low Impact Training
Mind and Body Fitness
Strength and Bodyweight Training

FITNESS AND TRAINING

MIND AND BODY FITNESS

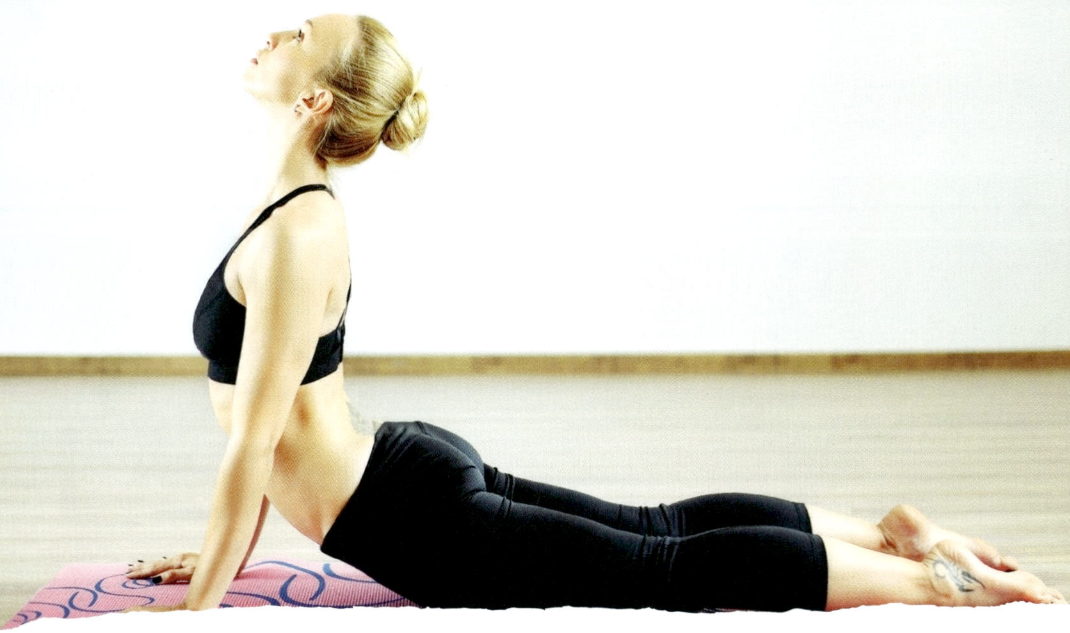

Cole Johnson

Mason Crest
Miami

Mason Crest
PO Box 221876
Hollywood, FL 33022
(866) MCP-BOOK (toll-free)
www.masoncrest.com

First printing
9 8 7 6 5 4 3 2 1
ISBN (hardback) 978-1-4222-4601-6
ISBN (series) 978-1-4222-4594-1
ISBN (ebook) 978-1-4222-7217-6

Library of Congress Cataloging-in-Publication Data

Names: Johnson, Cole, author.
Title: Mind and body Fitness / Cole Johnson.
Description: Hollywood, FL : Mason Crest, [2023] | Series: Fitness and training | Includes bibliographical references and index.
Identifiers: LCCN 2021056088 | ISBN 9781422246016 (hardcover) | ISBN 9781422272176 (ebook)
Subjects: LCSH: Mental health promotion—Juvenile literature. | Physical fitness—Psychological aspects—Juvenile literature. | Exercise—Psychological aspects—Juvenile literature. | Mind and body—Juvenile literature.
Classification: LCC RA790.53 .J65 2023 | DDC 613.7—dc23/eng/20220121
LC record available at https://lccn.loc.gov/2021056088

Developed and Produced by National Highlights, Inc.
Editor: Andrew Luke
Production: Crafted Content, LLC

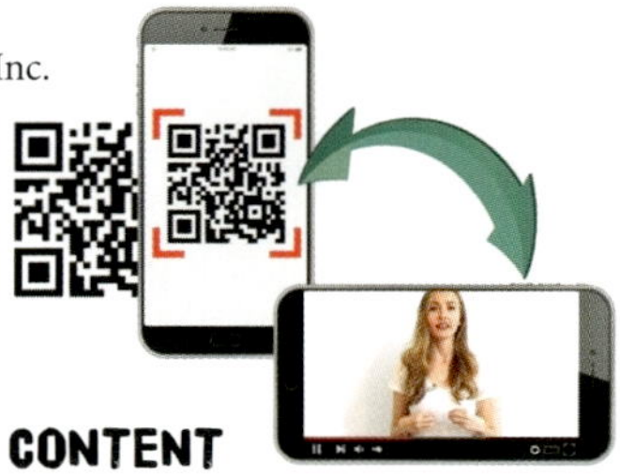

QR CODES AND LINKS TO THIRD-PARTY CONTENT

You may gain access to certain third-party content ("Third-Party Sites") by scanning and using the QR Codes that appear in this publication (the "QR Codes"). We do not operate or control in any respect any information, products, or services on such Third-Party Sites linked to by us via the QR Codes included in this publication, and we assume no responsibility for any materials you may access using the QR Codes. Your use of the QR Codes may be subject to terms, limitations, or restrictions set forth in the applicable terms of use or otherwise established by the owners of the Third-Party Sites. Our linking to such Third-Party Sites via the QR Codes does not imply an endorsement or sponsorship of such Third-Party Sites or the information, products, or services offered on or through the Third-Party Sites, nor does it imply an endorsement or sponsorship of this publication by the owners of such Third-Party Sites.

CONTENTS

KEY ICONS TO LOOK FOR

WORDS TO UNDERSTAND: These words, with their easy-to-understand definitions, will increase readers' understanding of the text while building vocabulary skills.

SIDEBARS: This boxed material within the main text allows readers to build knowledge, gain insights, explore possibilities, and broaden their perspectives by weaving together additional information to provide realistic and holistic perspectives.

EDUCATIONAL VIDEOS: Readers can view videos by scanning our QR codes, providing them with additional educational content to supplement the text.

TEXT-DEPENDENT QUESTIONS: These questions send the reader back to the text for more careful attention to the evidence presented there.

RESEARCH PROJECTS: Readers are pointed toward areas of further inquiry connected to each chapter. Suggestions are provided for projects that encourage deeper research and analysis.

SERIES GLOSSARY OF KEY TERMS: This back-of-the-book glossary contains terminology used throughout this series. Words found here increase the reader's ability to read and comprehend higher-level books and articles in this field.

WORDS TO UNDERSTAND

endorphins—peptides released by the brain that, among other functions, reduce perception of pain and induce feelings of euphoria

Centers for Disease Control and Prevention (CDC)—a U.S. government agency responsible for developing and applying disease prevention and control initiatives, environmental health, health promotion, and health education activities

National Institute of Mental Health (NIH)—the lead United States government agency for research on mental disorders.

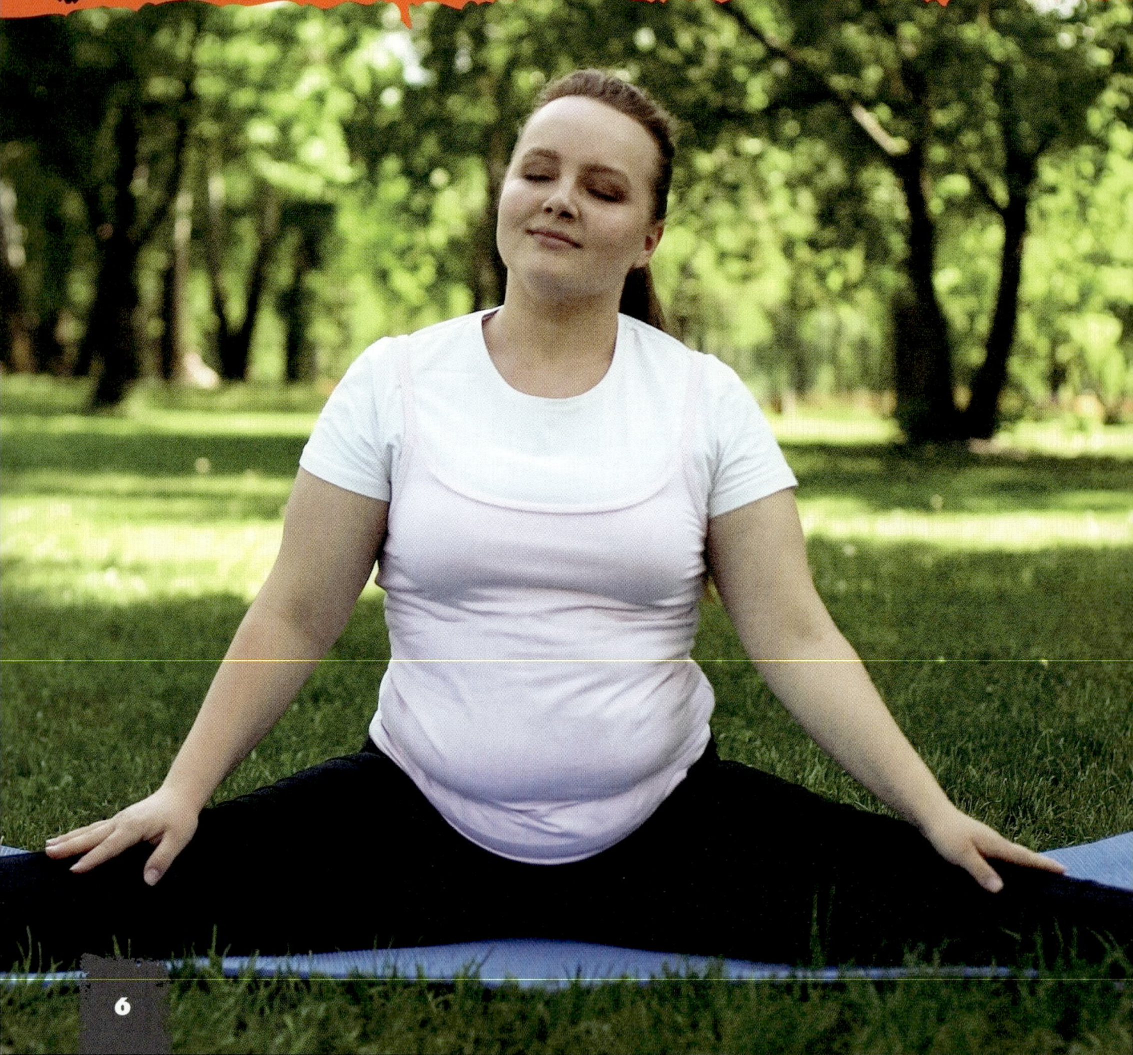

CHAPTER 1
FITNESS IS MORE THAN A PHYSICAL PURSUIT

When considering the term "fitness," the first things that probably come to your mind are activities like going to the gym, maintaining a healthy body weight, and drinking plenty of water. All of these variables are, without a doubt, integral parts of what it means to be fit. Physical fitness is strongly emphasized in our society today, primarily for its physiological benefits. Unfortunately, many other beneficial factors have also become prevalent for the wrong reasons all of the sudden.

In case you are unaware of just how sedentary we have become as a population, according to the most recent data collected by the **Centers for Disease Control and Prevention**, in 2018, approximately 42 percent of the U.S. population was considered obese. This phenomenon is unrivaled by any other period in time since this type of data has been reported. If simply stating the percentage of obese individuals living in the United States today does not do the issue enough justice, let's use raw numbers. In 2018, there were just 327 million people living in the United States. This means that more than 137 million of these individuals were obese!

As you can see, there is a legitimate reason that the need for regular exercise, and healthy dietary choices has become such a talking point. While being "fit" on a physical basis is one of most effective ways to ensure maximum quality of life and will be discussed in great detail throughout this book, there is another side to fitness that has seemingly taken a back seat to the obesity epidemic. This no-less-important variable in what constitutes overall fitness is mental health, and things are not looking so good in this area either.

THE BRAIN NEEDS EXERCISE TOO

Many people are familiar with how to become or remain physically fit by combining cardiovascular exercise with resistance training to improve vascular function as well as flexibility and strength. An exercise regimen that consistently includes some level of each of these is generally considered, along with a sensible diet, to be an effective whole-body approach to fitness. However, that conclusion leaves out an important part of the body…the brain.

It is a fact that the brain does get some benefit from physical exercise. A 2019 study published in the *Journal of the International Neuropsychological Society* found that exercise stimulates brain activity, especially in the brain's memory center.

Other studies have shown that it is possible (and advantageous) to exercise the brain without working up a sweat. Research shows that the brain wants to be challenged, which is why watching content on a screen for hours at a time is not just bad for the body.

Word games and board games that require deduction and strategy are good places to start. Dr. John Morley, professor of medicine at St. Louis University, suggests the following ideas as some other ways to exercise the brain to improve cognitive function:

1. Learn a list – it can be your favorite movies, albums or memes…just write down a list of them and try to memorize it in order.
2. Play it – learn to play a musical instrument. New and complex tasks that take time to master are the perfect brain challenge.
3. Say it – learn a new language. Studies have linked this challenging task to increased brain stimulation.
4. Throw your brain a curve ball – learn to play a different sport. If you play baseball, give tennis or golf a try. Something with a completely different set of rules and physical actions will keep your brain on its toes.
5. Concentrate to calculate – do math in your head. Ditch the calculator app the next time a situation arises requiring simple math. The extra few seconds it takes can mean extra benefits for the brain.

These exercises will challenge your brain and help keep it sharp.

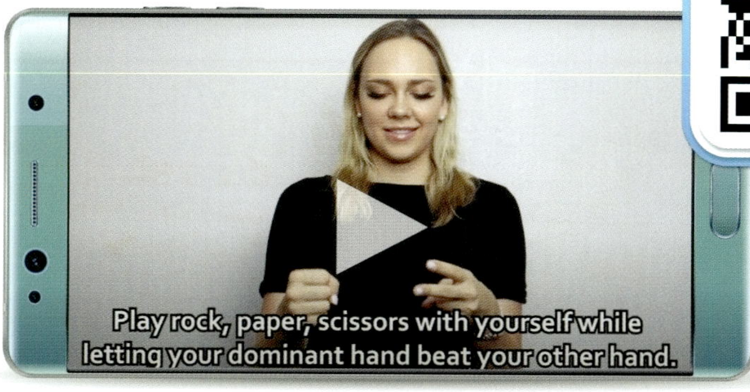
Play rock, paper, scissors with yourself while
letting your dominant hand beat your other hand.

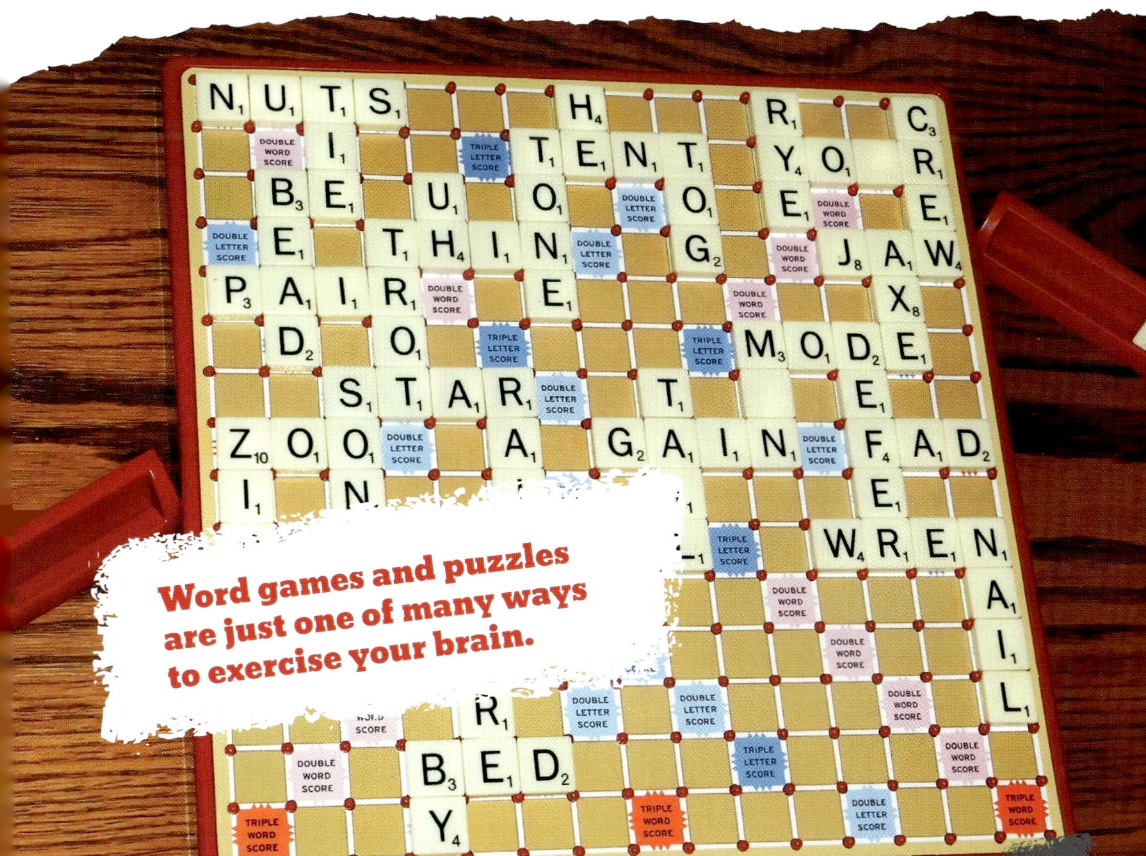

Word games and puzzles are just one of many ways to exercise your brain.

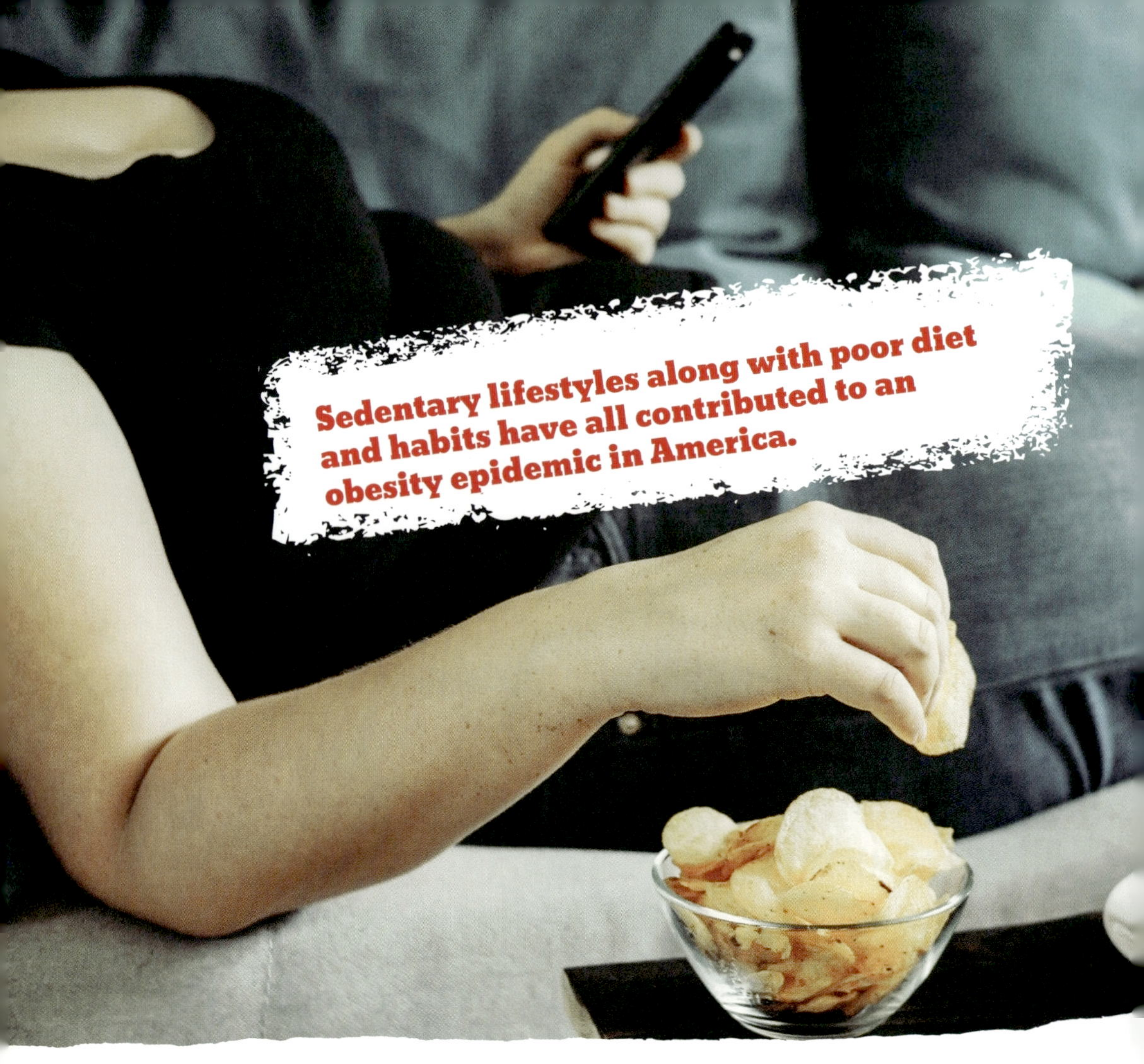
Sedentary lifestyles along with poor diet and habits have all contributed to an obesity epidemic in America.

OUR MENTAL HEALTH IS SUFFERING

With all of the discussion and attention being paid to the unfavorable state of physical fitness, it seems that the mental health of our population has been experiencing a relatively unnoticed decline as well. The **National Institute of Mental Health** has reported that as recently as 2017, a little more than seven percent of the U.S. population older than eighteen years of age has experienced at least one major depressive episode! This statistic only includes depression, leaving out a slew of other mental disorders that are on the rise, such as anxiety and chronic stress.

The reason for mental health failing to receive the attention it warrants today can probably be associated with a number of factors. The first and most obvious of these is that mental health problems are not usually obvious or visible. They are not something that is evident when passing someone on the street. When encountering an individual who is morbidly obese, there is not much left to question about the state of his or her physical fitness. On the contrary, mental illness typically fails to display anywhere near the observable warning signs or indications that something is amiss.

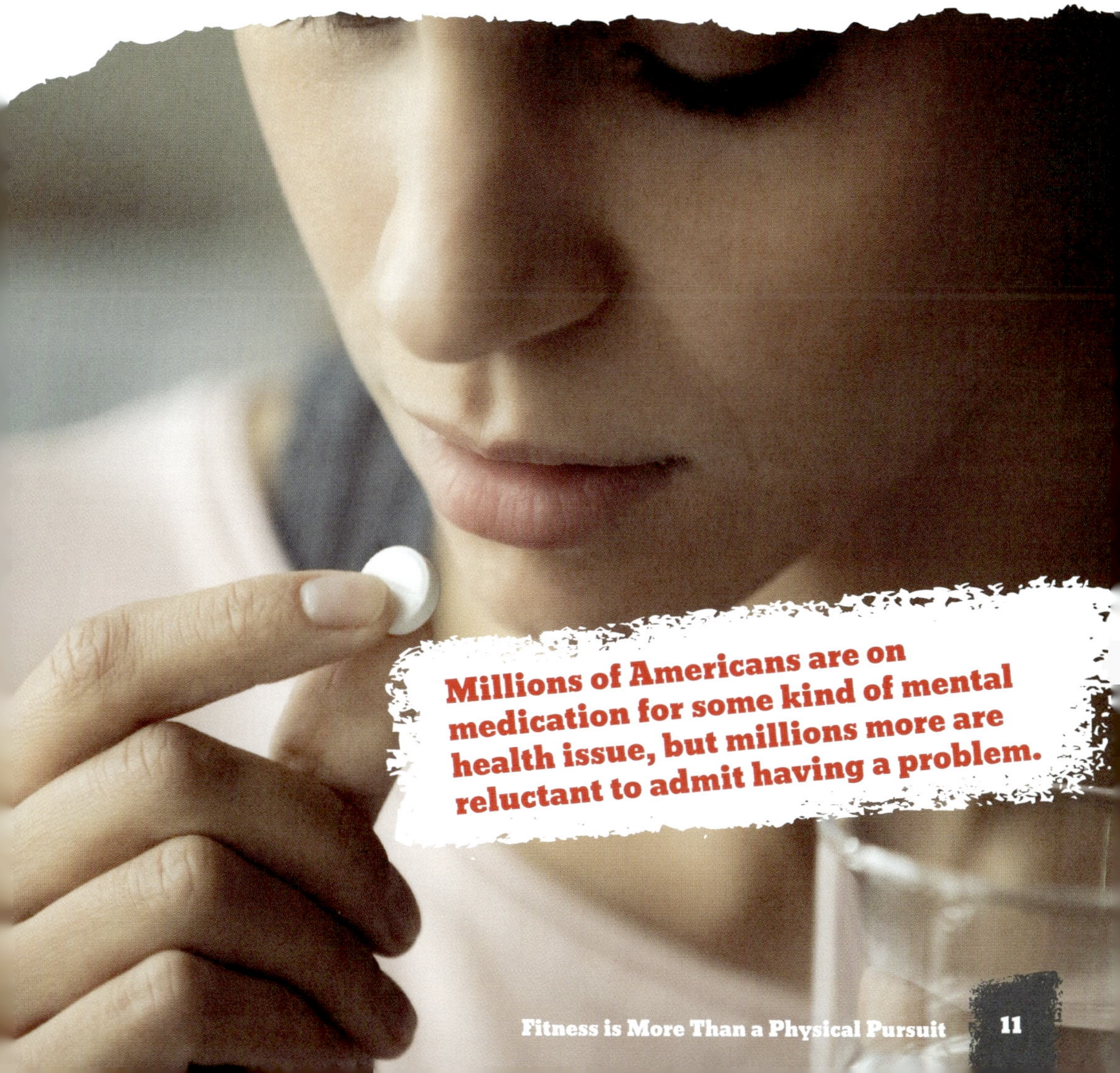

Millions of Americans are on medication for some kind of mental health issue, but millions more are reluctant to admit having a problem.

Another important and equally unfortunate reason that mental health disorders are not receiving enough attention is the fact that they are chronically underreported because people are reluctant to admit to problems. Somewhere along the way, it seems our society accepted obesity as a mainstream problem, one that can be openly discussed and worked on. For someone to admit any struggle with mental health, however, is largely taboo. The statistics available on the subject are already alarming, and these numbers only take into account the individuals seeking treatment for their issues.

ANTI-DEPRESSANTS ARE THE NEW ASPIRIN

The American Psychological Association reported that as of 2014, an astounding 64 percent of the population regularly took some form of antidepressant medication! As if that number alone doesn't put the issue into perspective, when this data was calculated in the year 1999, this number was a little more than seven percent. It is certainly no stretch to say that the statistics regarding obesity are disturbing, but perhaps equally as critical are those painting the picture of our mental health.

OUR CULTURAL DEFINITION OF FITNESS MUST BE REVISED

As human beings, we will always be inherently attracted to what we can see. When it comes to fitness, the impressive physiques adorning the containers in supplement stores and magazine pages are the shiny objects that draw us in. It is infinitely easier to sell you a workout program or product promising to give you six-pack abs than to convince you to spend your time and money on a technique that improves the way you view the world around you.

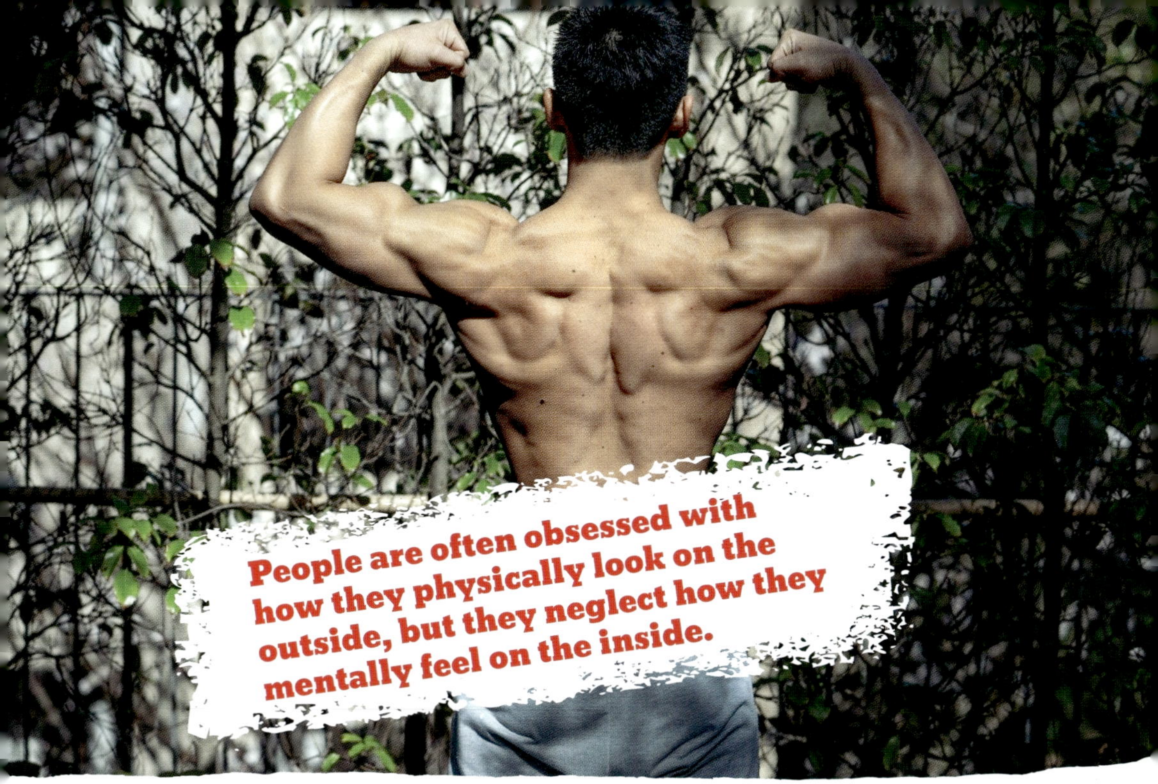
People are often obsessed with how they physically look on the outside, but they neglect how they mentally feel on the inside.

Don't think for a second that taking care of your body and aspiring to look great are not worthwhile goals. Your body is designed to move and perform in some incredible ways, and working hard to improve and maintain its function is of the utmost importance. In fact, a significant portion of this book will be dedicated to providing you with effective ways to improve your physical fitness.

However, this book goes beyond equipping you with knowledge to sustain your physical fitness. It also examines several really great methods to ensure your mental fitness is being attended to as well. You have probably heard of some of the well-known mental benefits of physical exercise, such as increased **endorphin** release, and there are a great many of them. Some of the ideas we break down will certainly build on the merits of physical activity as a way to fortify your body and mind. However, there will also be a much-needed portion of our discussion regarding methods and techniques designed to directly exercise your mind. Killing two birds with one stone is usually the way to go, but just like emphasizing your workout routine to build a particular muscle group, sometimes improving your mental fitness requires your full attention!

ENDORPHINS

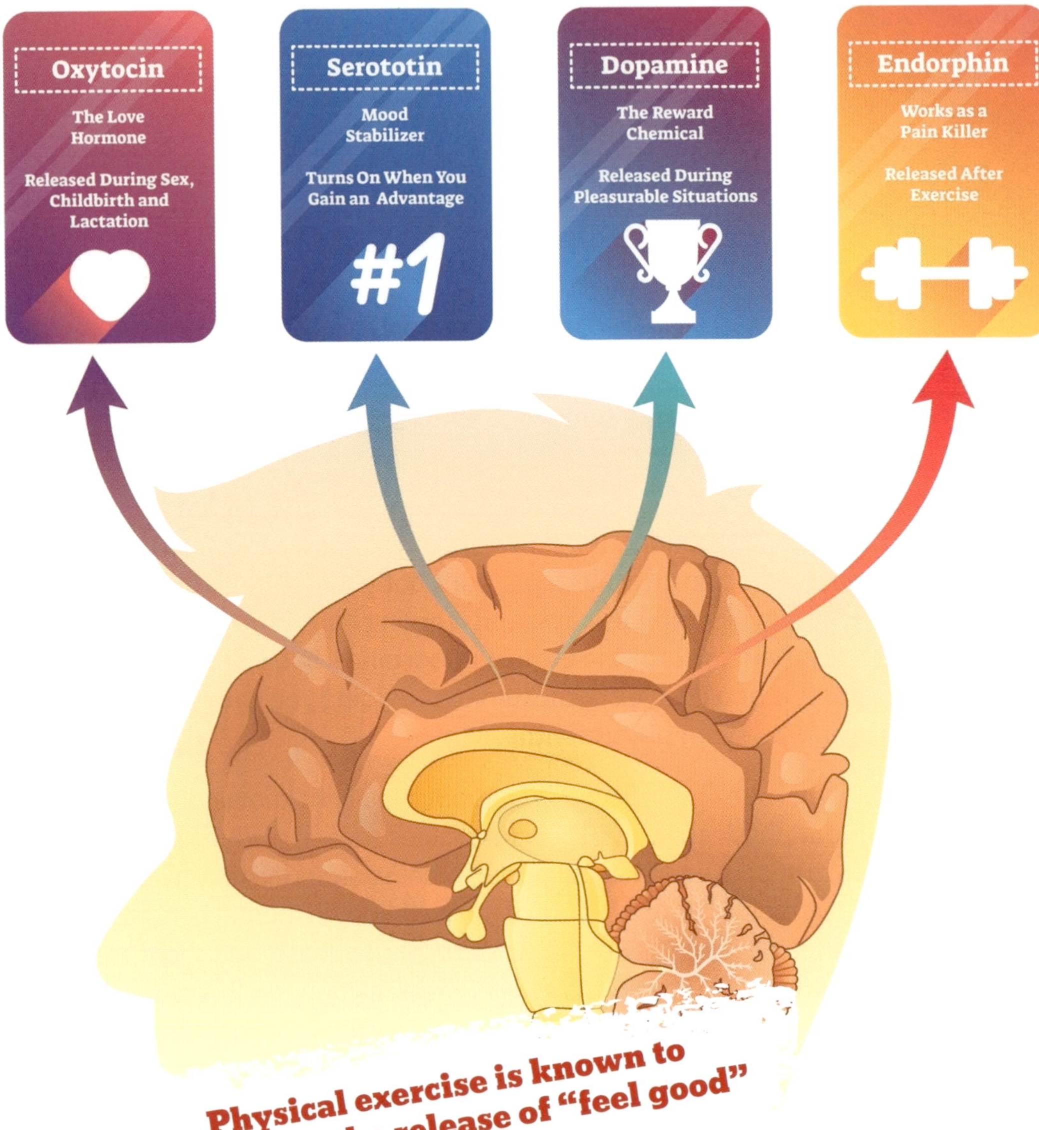

Physical exercise is known to trigger the release of "feel good" hormones in the brain.

Instead of completely erasing the definition of fitness you probably had in mind, think in terms of simply expanding on that definition. Being physically fit and maintaining a great physique will most certainly improve your life and the experiences you get to enjoy. You just need to realize there is more to the equation. Not only is it important to acknowledge that your mental fitness is an equally important component of what it means to be "fit," but also the relationship between physical and mental fitness is another topic that desperately needs to be addressed. These two variables have always gone hand-in-hand. If you want to really get the most out of everything life has to offer, making sure that your internal environment is being nourished right alongside your physical state is of utmost importance. As human beings, we are all incredibly complex and unique creatures. There is always more to someone than meets the eye.

ANOTHER CAR ANALOGY

For whatever reason, explaining certain situations using a car seems to be the way to go. Not to be cliché, but the analogy works great with the idea we are emphasizing here. Think of your physical health as the outside of the car. Everyone loves a shiny set of rims, sleek paint job, and freshly cleaned exterior. These things are great and definitely important. However, none of them matter much if the mechanical components of the car, the transmission, electronics, etc., are falling to pieces. Your mental health is the inner workings of the car that other people rarely see. Don't spend so much time working on your physique and physical fitness that you end up neglecting the equally important side of who you are—your mental health.

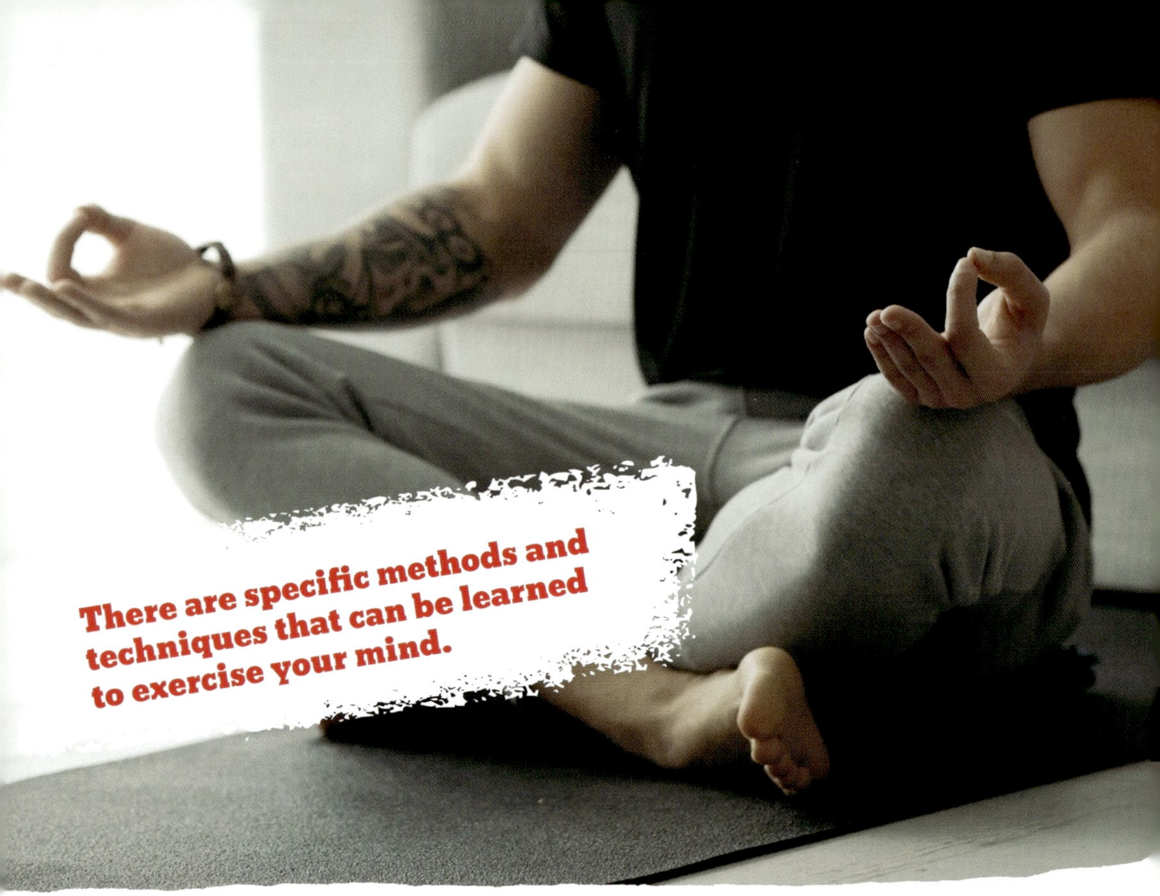

There are specific methods and techniques that can be learned to exercise your mind.

This video quickly and humorously portrays the way that our society takes physical health and fitness very seriously, while mental health issues are supposed to be handled by the individual suffering from them.

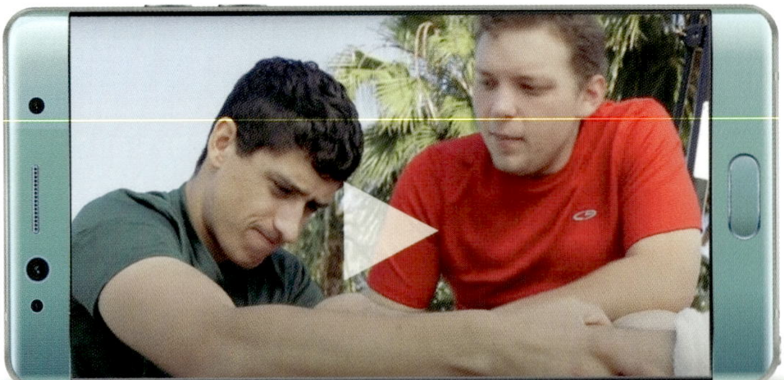

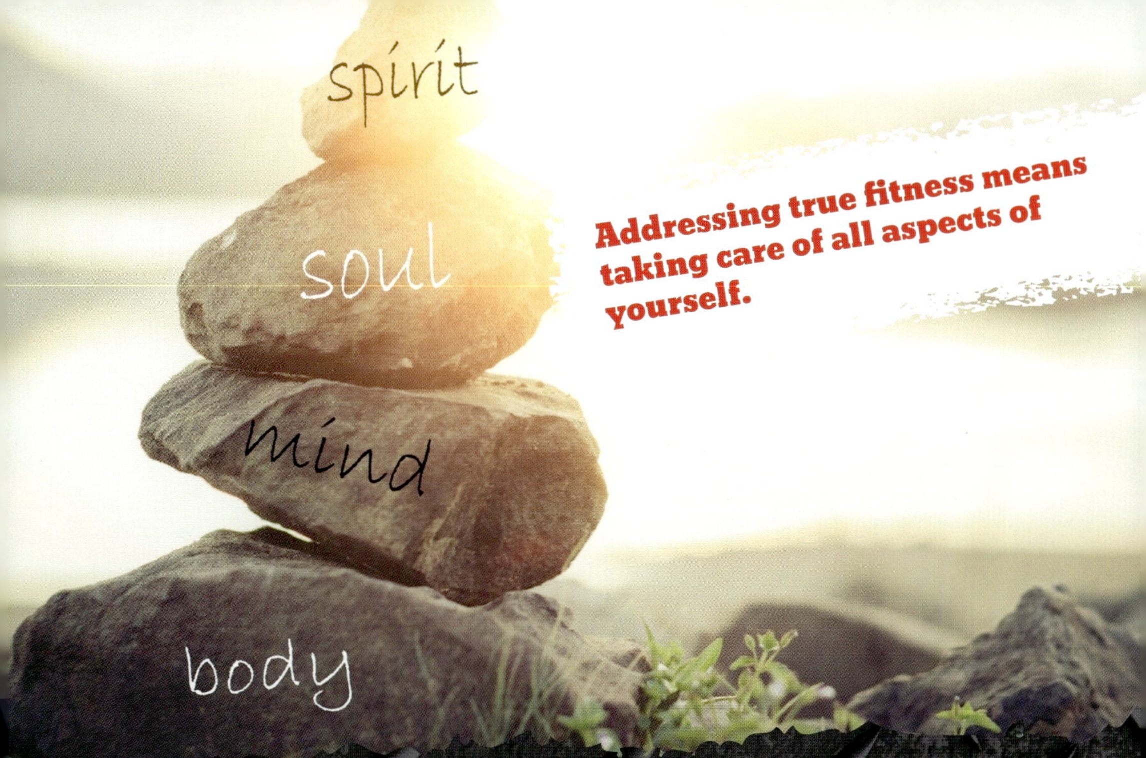

Addressing true fitness means taking care of all aspects of yourself.

TEXT-DEPENDENT QUESTIONS

1. According to the chapter, what is one primary reason that mental health often goes unnoticed when compared to physical health?
2. What is the percent increase in the number of individuals in the United States taking antidepressant medication from 1999 to 2014?
3. What is the general idea behind the word “fitness” in today’s society?

RESEARCH PROJECT

In this chapter, the significant percentage of the population dealing with depression was highlighted. However, alluding to the fact that many other mental disorders are also on the rise followed this. Think about another prevalent mental disorder, such as anxiety. Research to determine what percentage of our population is dealing with this issue? What has been the general trend regarding this disorder over the last decade? Detail your answers in a short paper.

WORDS TO UNDERSTAND

flow state—the mental state in which a person performing an activity is fully immersed in a feeling of energized focus, full involvement, and enjoyment in the process of the activity

interoception—the sense of the internal state of the body

mindfulness—the practice of maintaining a nonjudgmental state of heightened or complete awareness of one's thoughts, emotions, or experiences on a moment-to-moment basis

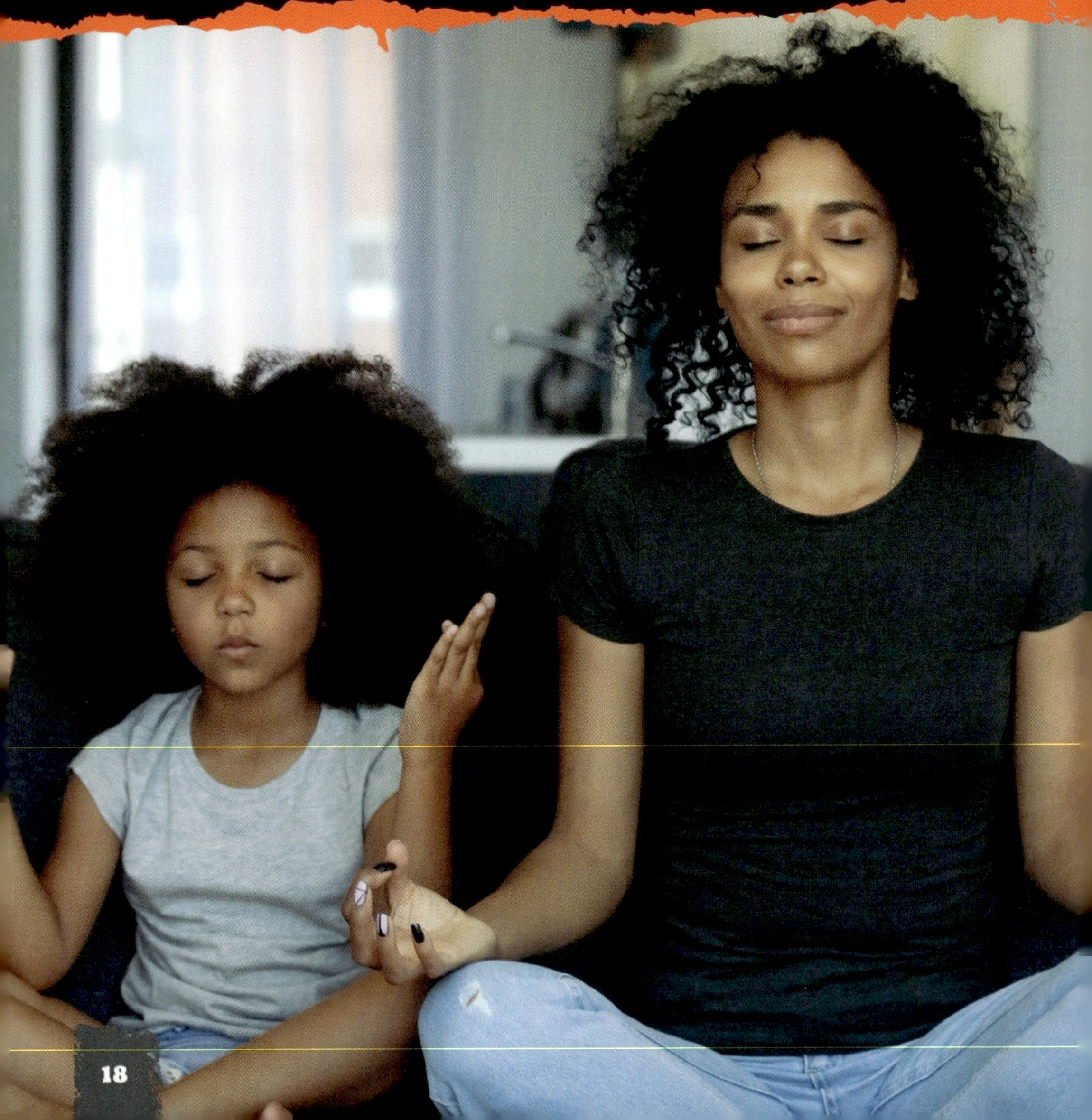

CHAPTER 2
SPECIFIC EXERCISES TO ENHANCE MENTAL FITNESS

As previously mentioned, there is nowhere near enough emphasis in our society on how to nurture and maintain a strong sense of mental fitness. While a large portion of the content provided here will be focused on ways in which to exercise your physical and mental states simultaneously, it is imperative that we first describe a few techniques aimed directly at the mind.

There are many important terms and keywords that, unfortunately, lose their significance and merit because they are used again and again to the point of becoming a cliché. **Mindfulness** is one such term. This word perfectly encapsulates everything that our world today is not. The amount of stimuli begging for our attention from many directions, combined with our restless minds that never stop ruminating over past events and future possibilities, has created a society in which being totally aware of the present moment can be difficult.

A person's lifetime is a relatively short period broken down into moments that come and go, never being able to be relived. A life spent living in the past or present, not the moment that is right in front of you, lends to the possibility of missing some of those key moments, or at least not appreciating them fully.

Here are three great exercises that, when performed correctly, focus on the present and induce a much-needed sense of mindfulness. These exercises are designed to allow your focus to shift from a place of being overwhelmed by the immensity of your external environment to a place of **interoception**. While you may have had brief periods in your life when you felt truly in the moment, entirely focused on the exact place and time, interoception is different.

BODY SCAN MEDITATION

This form of mindfulness exercise is a fantastic way to get into a sort of **flow state**, in which the world around you shrinks to the size of your body. The name of this technique, body scan meditation, is important. During this exercise, you will be centering your awareness on each individual part of your body. All too often we seem to have the unconscious sense that something is a little off in our body, but we are too consumed in the craziness of day-to-day life that we rarely even take the time to slow down and pinpoint where the issue is! Body scan meditation is a way to pay attention to yourself as a whole through precise breathing and attention shifts.

Before going into the specifics behind how to practice body scan meditation, it is important to point out the significant amount of research supporting this technique as an effective way to reduce stress and mental fatigue. A report published in *Mindfulness,* a research journal dedicated to information regarding its namesake, researchers sought to compare the effects of body scan meditation on several key biological markers known to increase during periods of stress or anxiety (namely cortisol) versus simply listening to an audiobook. This study divided 47 subjects into two groups. Each day for a period of eight weeks, one group performed a 20-minute body scan meditation, while the other simply listened to an audiobook for the same length of time. At the conclusion of the study, the subjects practicing body scan meditation universally experienced decreases in cortisol as well as a significant reduction in their reported levels of stress. Interestingly, the subjects in the audio book group actually saw an increase in both of these variables!

To implement this technique into your day, plan on setting aside 5–20 minutes of time where you are able to be alone in a relatively quiet environment. You can either lie down or assume a seated, relaxed position. Begin taking slow, deep breaths until you have established a comfortable breathing pattern. To begin the scan, bring all of your attention to your feet, noticing any sensation or discomfort that may be present. Hold your focus on this area for a minute or so while you

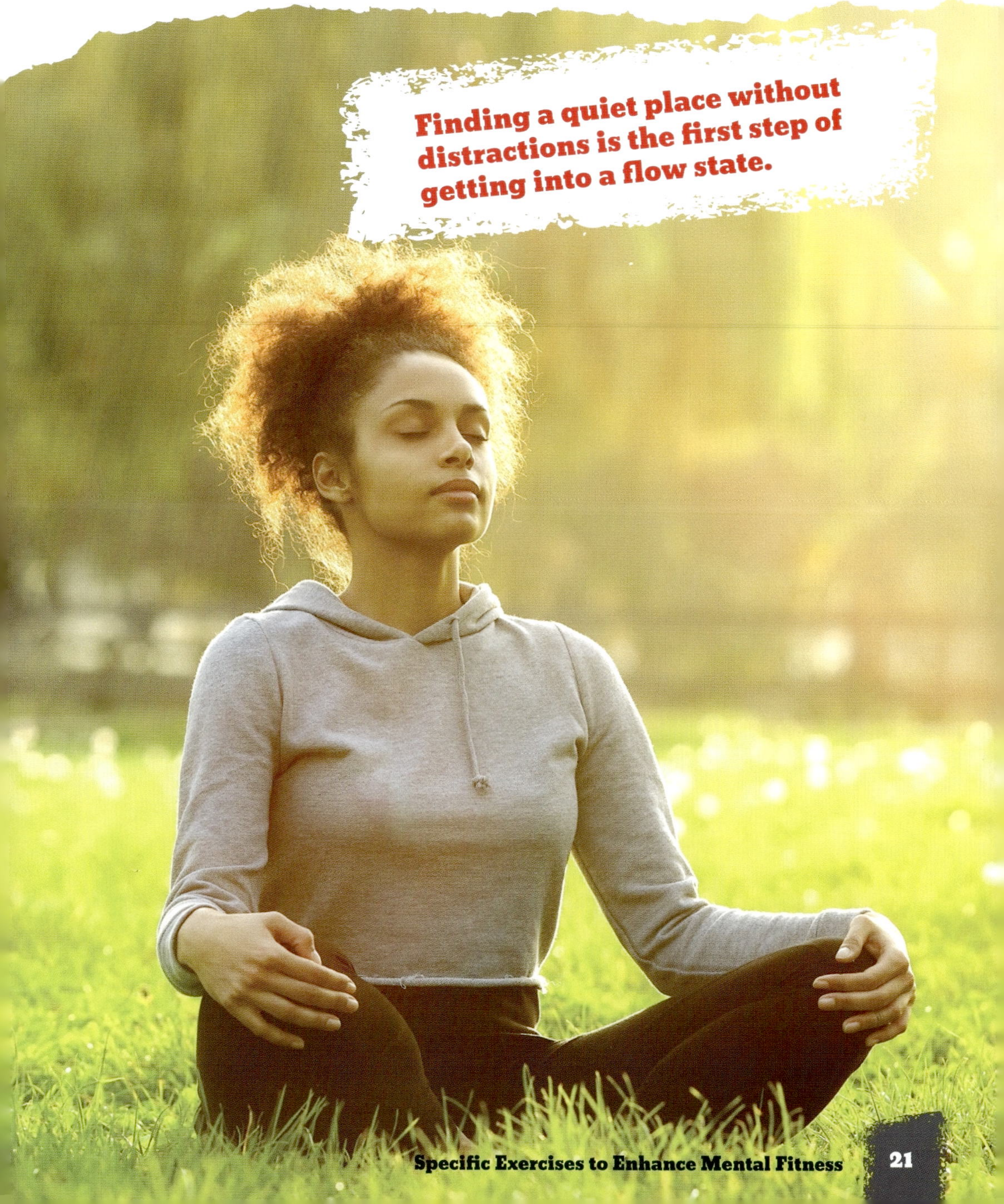
Finding a quiet place without distractions is the first step of getting into a flow state.

This video provides a great example of a quick and effective body scan meditation that can easily be included in some part of your day.

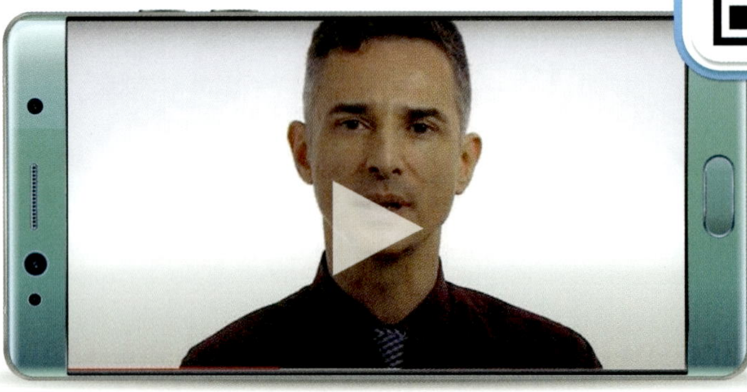

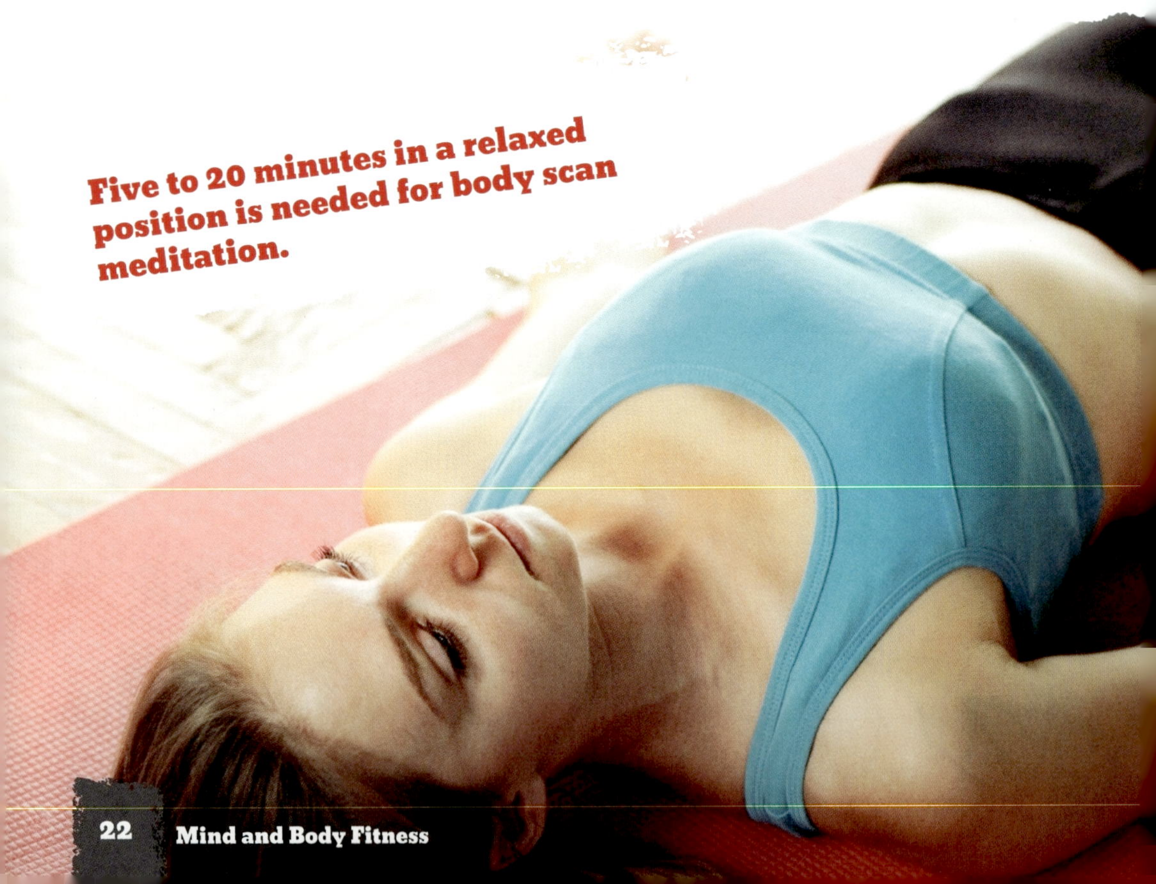

Five to 20 minutes in a relaxed position is needed for body scan meditation.

continue to breathe deeply. You will then move upwards toward your shins and knees, giving these areas your full attention and once again taking the time to fully notice any sense of pressure or discomfort. This exact process will then continue to migrate up your body until the top of your head is fully scanned and accounted for. When you are finished, take a few deeper, cleansing breaths and open your eyes.

MINDFUL BREATHING

As simple as it sounds, centering your entire thought process and attention on simply breathing is another extremely beneficial way to exercise your mental fitness. The fact that this is considered an exercise for human beings today says a lot about our current state.

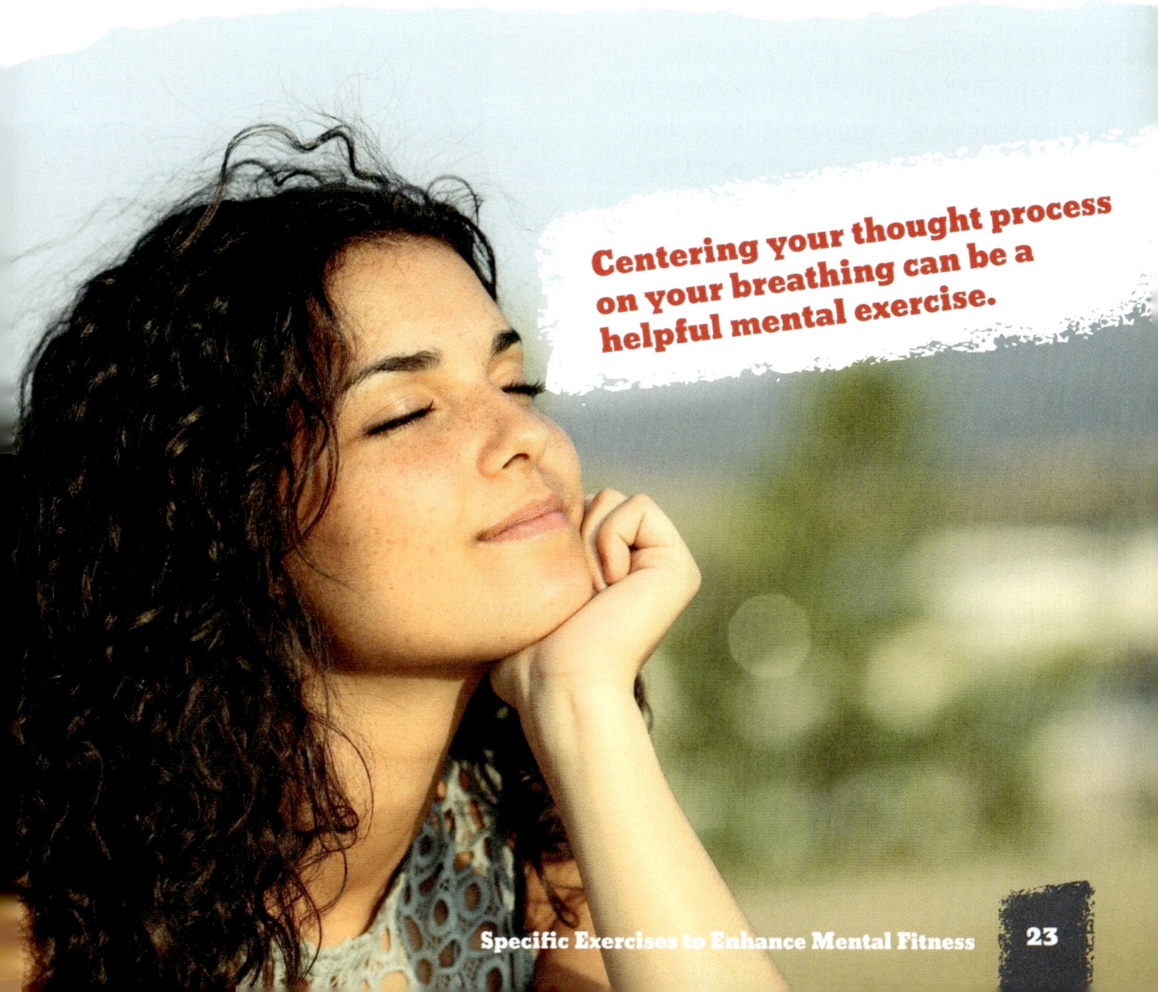
Centering your thought process on your breathing can be a helpful mental exercise.

Mindful breathing is another extremely simple way to remove yourself from the static and attention-grabbing bells and whistles everywhere you look. The *Journal of Clinical Psychiatry* describes a research experiment in which 93 individuals diagnosed with generalized anxiety disorder were asked to participate in either a mindfulness breathing routine or a stress management education course for an eight-week period. Before and after their participation in either intervention, all subjects completed primary outcome measures commonly used to quantify anxiety. At the end of the eight-week post-testing period, the subjects who adhered to a mindfulness breathing routine saw their scores decrease significantly over the other group in three of the four outcome measures.

SHORTENING YOUR GAZE

As you go through each day, virtually every part of your routine involves looking outwardly. This outward gaze can be short, such as checking social media accounts on your phone, or it might be long, as you notice a traffic light about to turn red half a mile up the road. These are just a couple of hundreds of examples that replay over and over each day. Consider this: when is the last time you looked inwardly? From time to time, it is important to reverse your usual outward gaze in order to notice your own body and the ever-present happenings within yourself.

Practicing a mindful breathing routine looks a lot like the body scan method we previously discussed. After finding a calm and quiet location, sit in a relaxed position. This can be on the floor or in a comfortable chair. Once again, close your eyes and begin to establish a pattern of deep breathing. What you will most likely find is that the second you intentionally turn your thoughts to your breath, your mind wants to run wild with a million other thoughts. This is perfectly fine and an absolutely normal occurrence. When these thoughts come, the

Mindful breathing is not about blocking out your thoughts, but rather allowing them to pass through your mind unchecked.

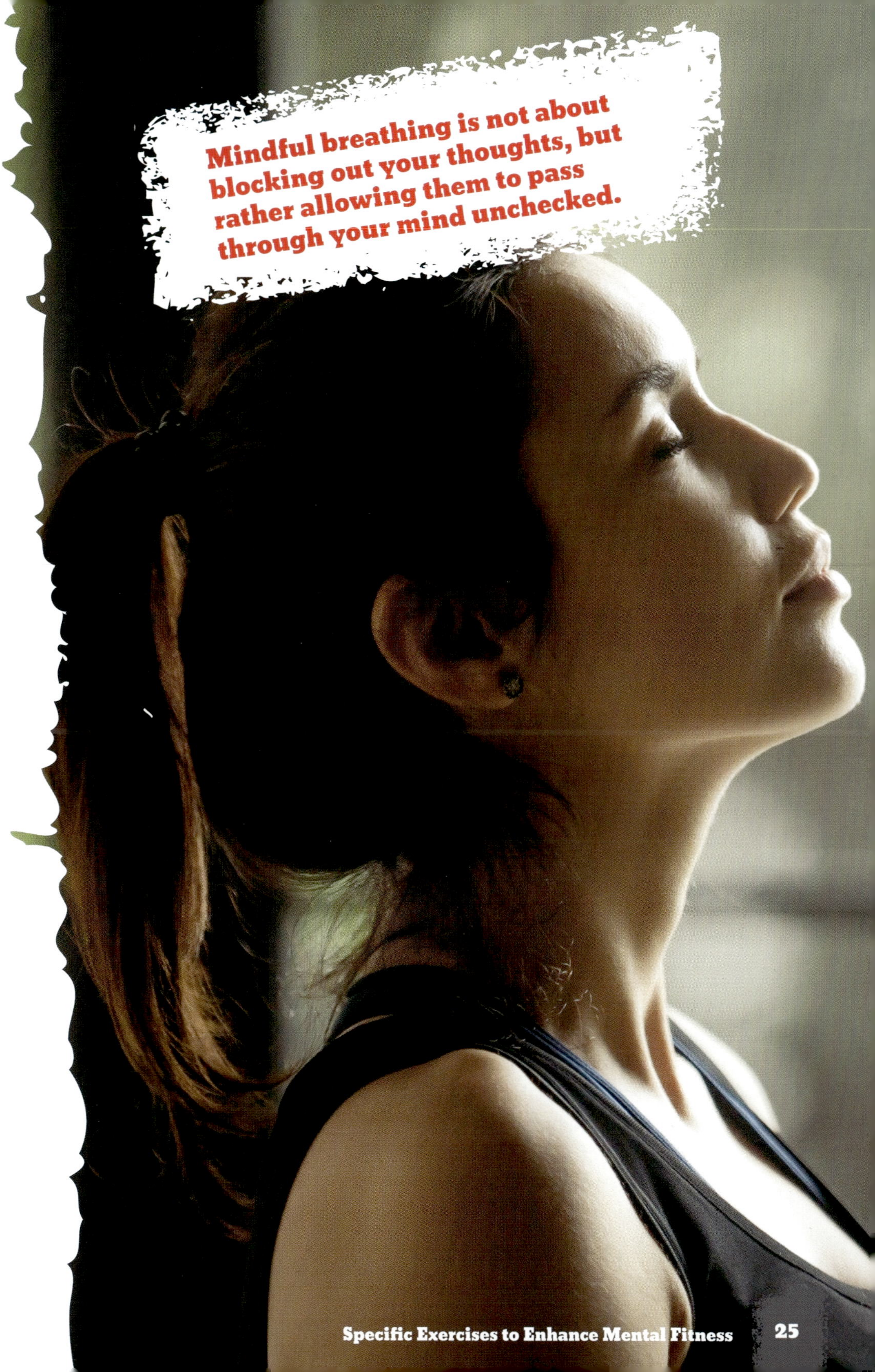

trick is to avoid resisting them. As you continue to focus on your breathing, think of your mind as nothing but a place for thoughts to pass through. During this exercise you are not labeling your thoughts as good or bad, you are simply acknowledging they are there before letting them dissolve. As with any exercise, you will struggle with this at first. This is why we are using the term mental "fitness". As you continue to practice and refine this technique, you will notice that your ability to maintain a calming breathing pattern while simultaneously resisting the urge to grab onto your thoughts will greatly improve.

APPRECIATE THE LITTLE THINGS

With all the noise and clutter going on around us seemingly all the time, it is so easy to become consumed in the fray. However, how much would any of these things matter the second you ran out of oxygen? While this sounds extreme, consider the question. How then, if breathing is something that we absolutely require at all times to stay alive, do we rarely if ever take the time to focus on it? Sitting still and making an effort to enjoy the gift of an invigorating gulp of oxygen is a simple activity that can help you attain a state of mindfulness.

EXPANDING AWARENESS MEDITATION

This mindfulness exercise may seem quite ironic at first. We have emphasized how important it can be to leave the noise and confusion of the world around you to focus on your own presence and the moment at hand. As you read the description of how to perform this exercise, it may seem ironic that you are asked to notice not only where you are in that moment but also expand your thoughts to the room, the building, the city, and so on. The difference between expanding awareness meditation and your usual perspective of the world around you is that during the exercise, you are gradually and methodically expanding your focus at a controlled rate. This allows you to precisely consider any problem

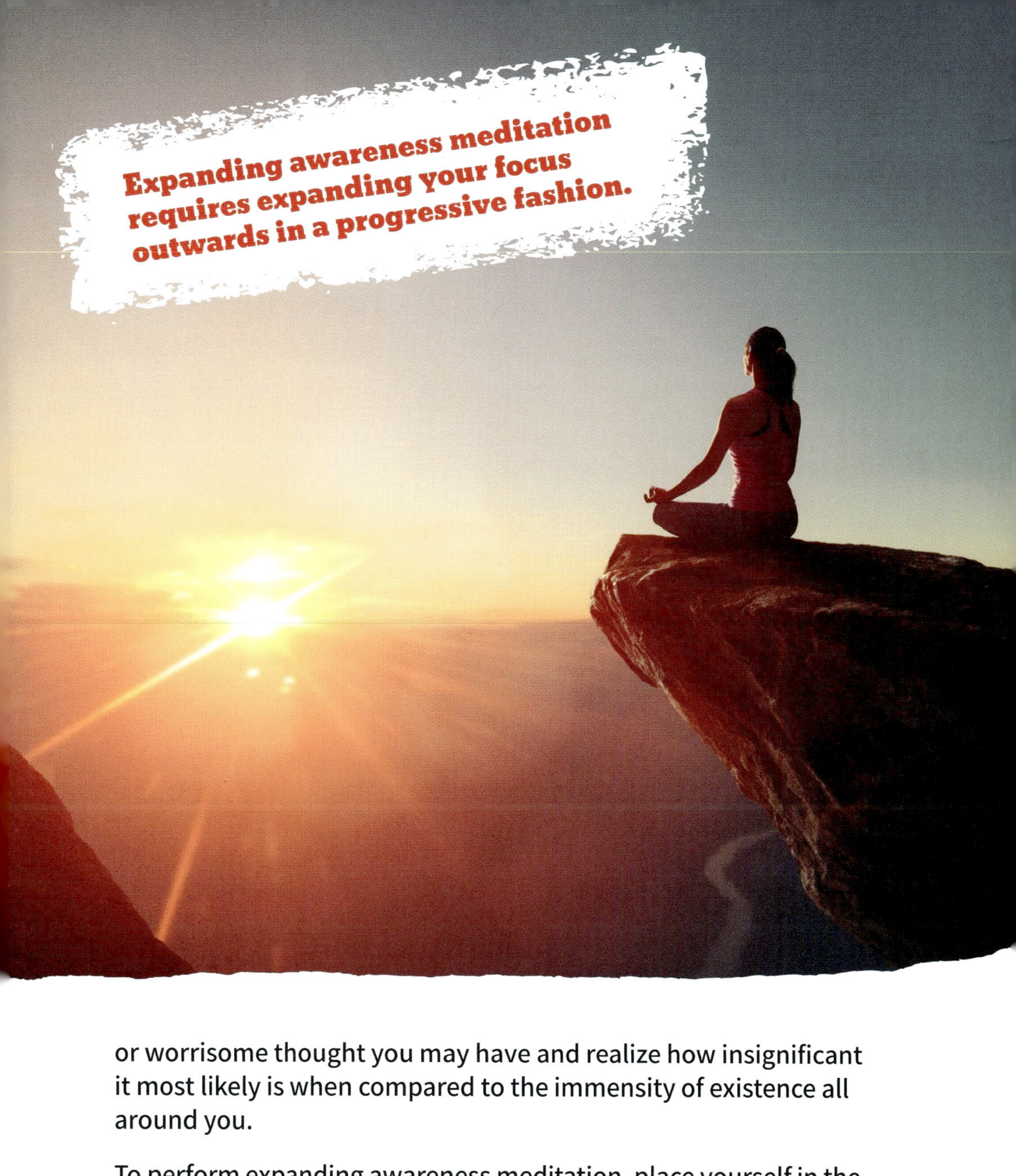
Expanding awareness meditation
requires expanding your focus
outwards in a progressive fashion.

or worrisome thought you may have and realize how insignificant it most likely is when compared to the immensity of existence all around you.

To perform expanding awareness meditation, place yourself in the same type of environment as previously described. Once you find a comfortable position, close your eyes. As you breath peacefully, start to imagine your body as the only thing in existence. Think about any sensations you are feeling, any thoughts going through your mind. Next, think about your body and the room you are located in at that

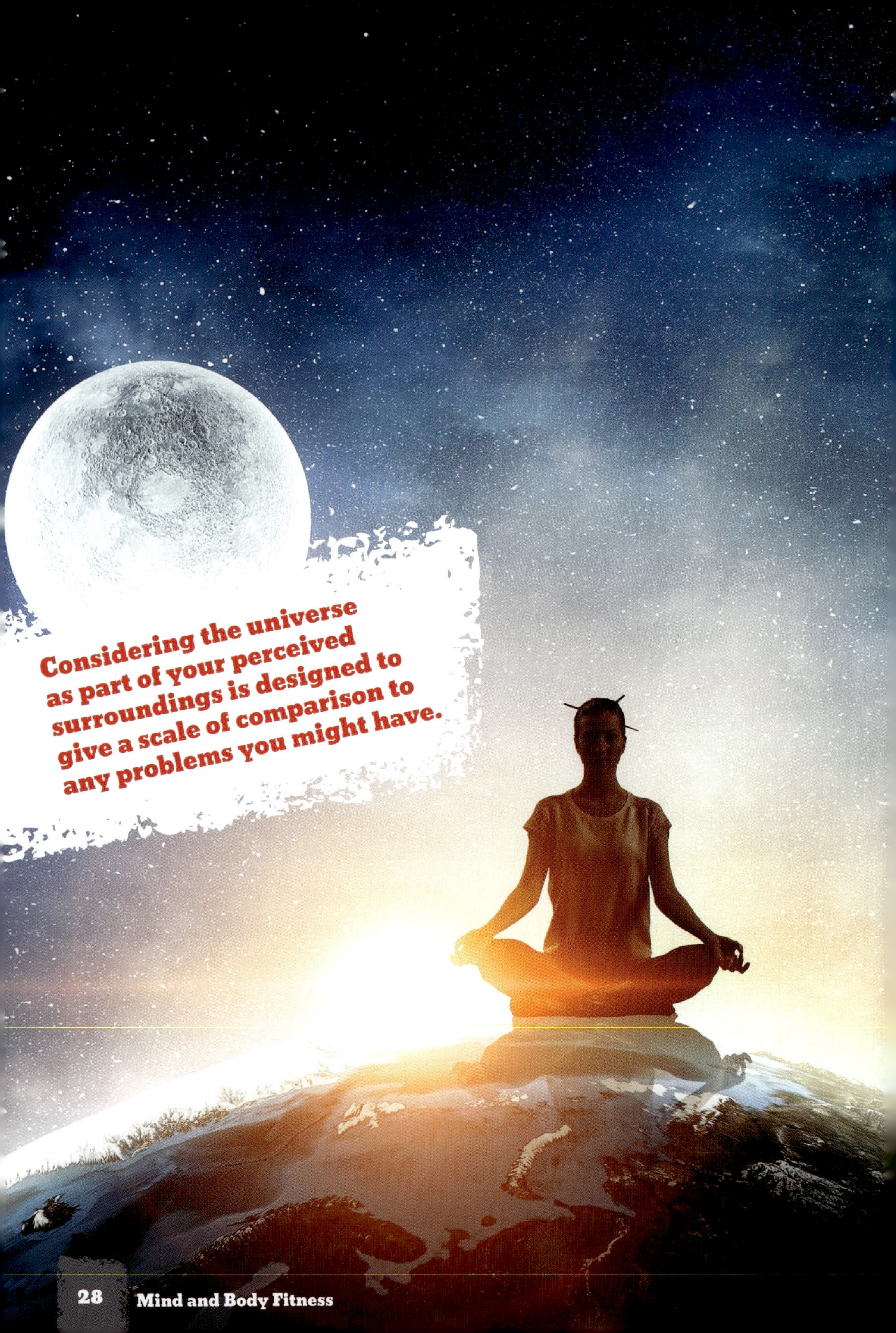

Considering the universe as part of your perceived surroundings is designed to give a scale of comparison to any problems you might have.

moment. Picture those four walls as if they contained the entire universe. As you continue to breath and sit comfortably, begin to let this universe grow very gradually. Think about the building you are in, then the street, city, and so on. As this mental universe continues to expand, think about the country, continent, and Earth itself. Once your perceived surroundings have expanded to include the actual universe itself, stay there for a moment. Go back to the issue or discomfort plaguing your mind at the start of this exercise. How small does it now seem? To conclude, enjoy a few more gentle breaths before opening your eyes.

TEXT-DEPENDENT QUESTIONS

1. What is one similarity attributed to all three forms of mental exercise discussed in this chapter?
2. What is the general flow of attention during most forms of body scan meditation?
3. How is expanded awareness meditation different from our usual way of perceiving the external environment?

RESEARCH PROJECT

Research the different types of mindfulness exercises. Take components from each one that you find appealing then create your own mindfulness exercise program. Detail how often it should be done and for how long. Be sure to give your new program a unique name.

WORDS TO UNDERSTAND

endogenous—having an internal cause or origin
muscle adhesion—scar tissue that develops in a muscle that often causes tenderness and reduced range of motion
neurogenesis—the growth and development of nervous system tissue

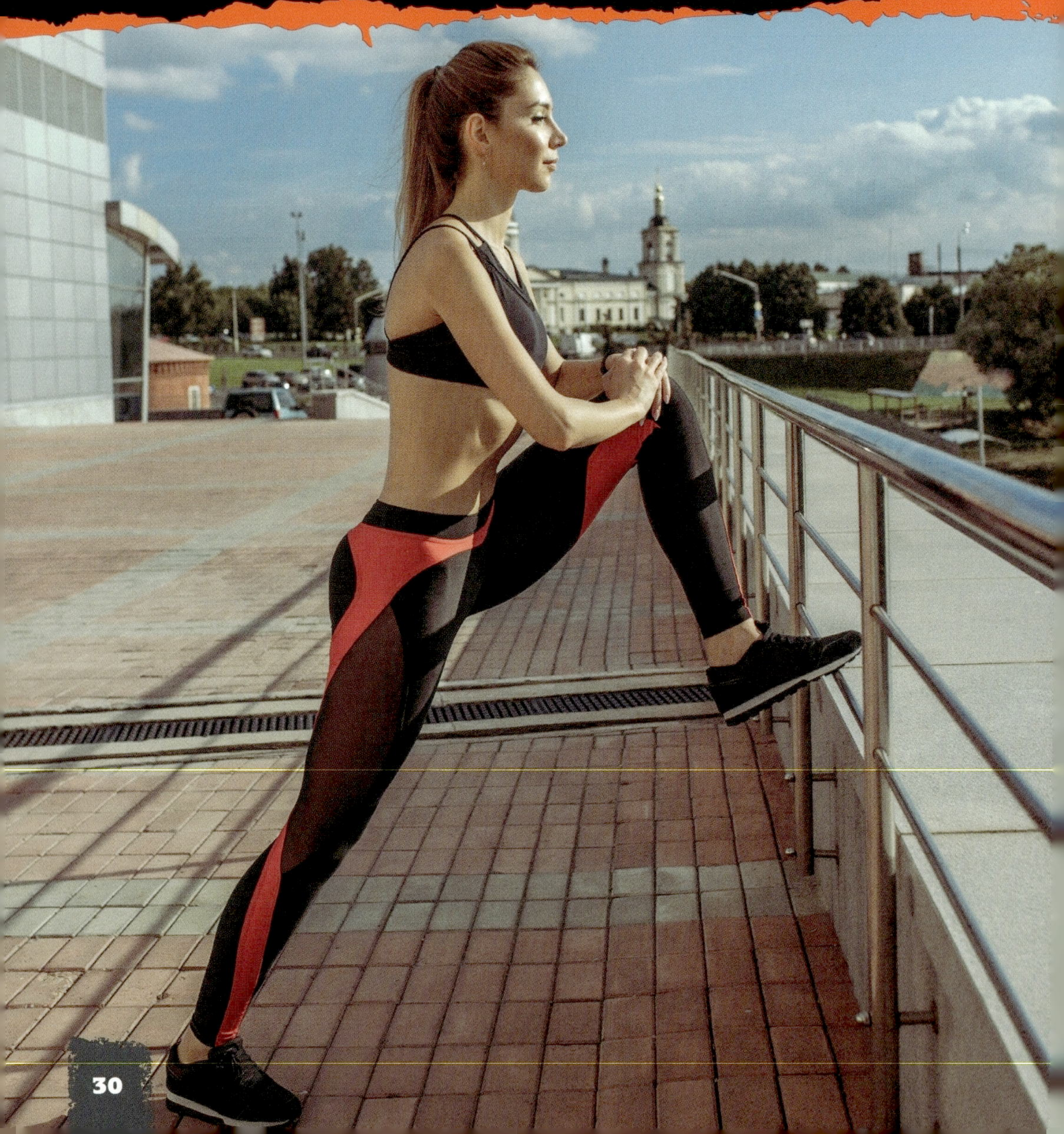

CHAPTER 3
HOW EXERCISE BENEFITS MENTAL HEALTH

Although your mind and body can certainly be exercised individually through things like going to the gym or enjoying a meditation session, physical exercise in general is fantastic for your mental health. Before getting into exercise methods that are supported by the research to improve physical and mental fitness, it is important to understand the "how" behind the concept.

Exercising and performing challenging physical activities have long been known to improve mental health. While many of us probably do not go to the gym, group exercise class, or running trail intending to nourish our minds, this still occurs even as we visualize the physical goals we wish to accomplish. With the knowledge that physical exercise is working its magic on your mind and body simultaneously, as well as understanding the reasons why, your motivation to continue taking care of yourself, your *entire* self, will certainly gain some traction!

EXERCISE AND DEPRESSION

New research continues to reveal how prevalent depression is in our country, and there are an enormous number of individuals taking antidepressant medication. While this medication is, no doubt, helpful for a large portion of people diagnosed with depression and should absolutely be utilized if it provides some relief, there are also some unwanted side effects (as if often the case with any medication).

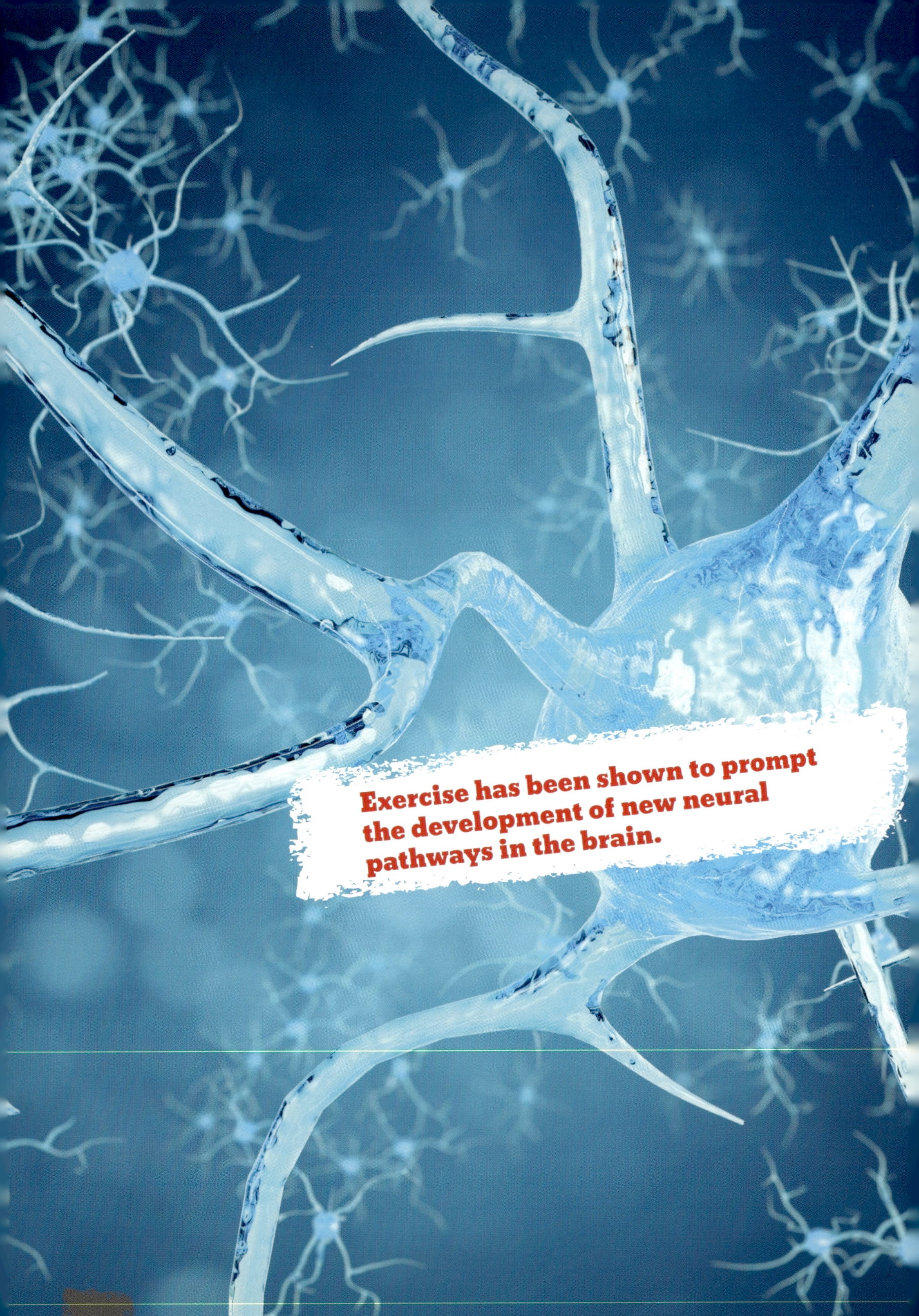

Exercise has been shown to prompt the development of new neural pathways in the brain.

There are quite a few popular ways of dealing with depression from a non-pharmacological perspective, and exercise is at the top of this list. Research after research study supports how getting enough exercise, in any form, can both prevent and alleviate depression. These benefits are thought to occur for a number of reasons. First of all, exercise increases the flow of oxygen-rich blood throughout your entire body, including the brain. This increased supply of oxygen and nutrients is necessary to both nourish the brain as a whole as well as to detoxify the brain through the flushing of waste products. Furthermore, exercise is known to increase "feel-good" hormones in the brain such as serotonin. This effect is somewhat compounded by the fact that frequent exercise causes **neurogenesis** in your brain, which basically builds new pathways as you develop new habits and activities. As your brain begins to build this new reward system pathway that is stimulated by exercise, you not only receive an increased surge of serotonin more consistently, but the old neural pathways (bad habits, negative self-talk, etc.) must be pruned away to make room for these new ones.

(UN) SHORTEN YOUR GAZE

As seen in earlier chapters, as far as your mental fitness is concerned, it is necessary to draw your focus in. Really taking the time to notice your body and breathing is a great way to practice mindfulness. Ironically, sometimes exercise is great for our minds for the exact opposite approach. When you are busting your tail during a really hard workout, you do not have time to dwell on the troublesome thought that has been running through your mind all day. Getting into your headspace is very beneficial in the appropriate context. Exercise pulls you out of your own head when you need it.

The *Journal of the American Medical Association Psychiatry* was able to use data available from a whopping 611,583 participants to observe any correlation between levels of physical activity and depression. What they found was not surprising. Even when comparing the data from such

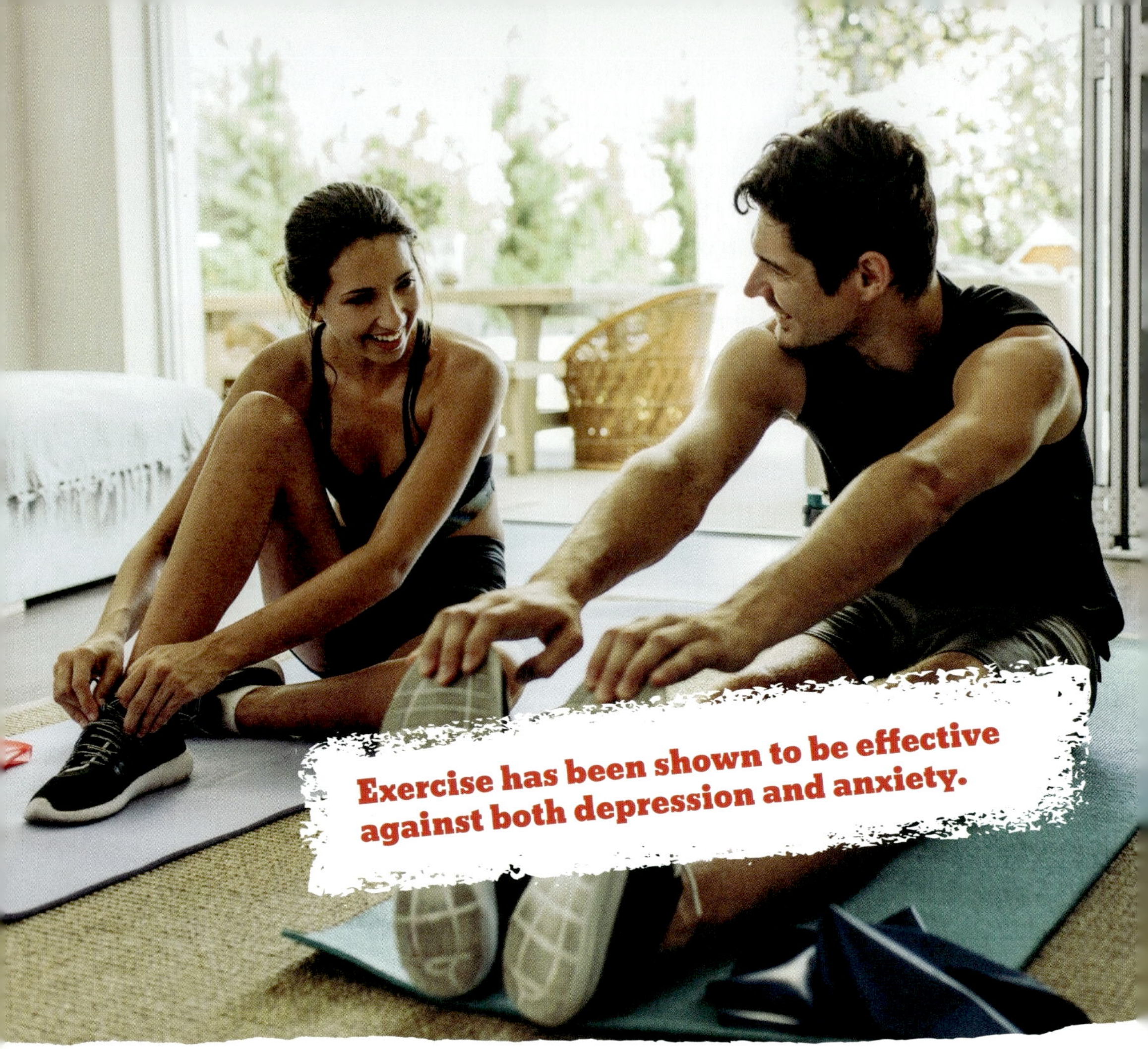
Exercise has been shown to be effective against both depression and anxiety.

a large number of subjects, the conclusion was that increased levels of physical activity displayed a strong negative correlation with depression and depression-like symptoms.

EXERCISE AND ANXIETY

Exercise is a great tool against anxiety for many of the same reasons it works so well against depression. Many of the biological responses useful at mitigating symptoms of depression, such as increased serotonin levels, work equally as well in reducing anxiety. There is another aspect of exercise that works particularly well in reducing what

Exercise forces you to focus on the movements you need to make rather than the things you are worried about.

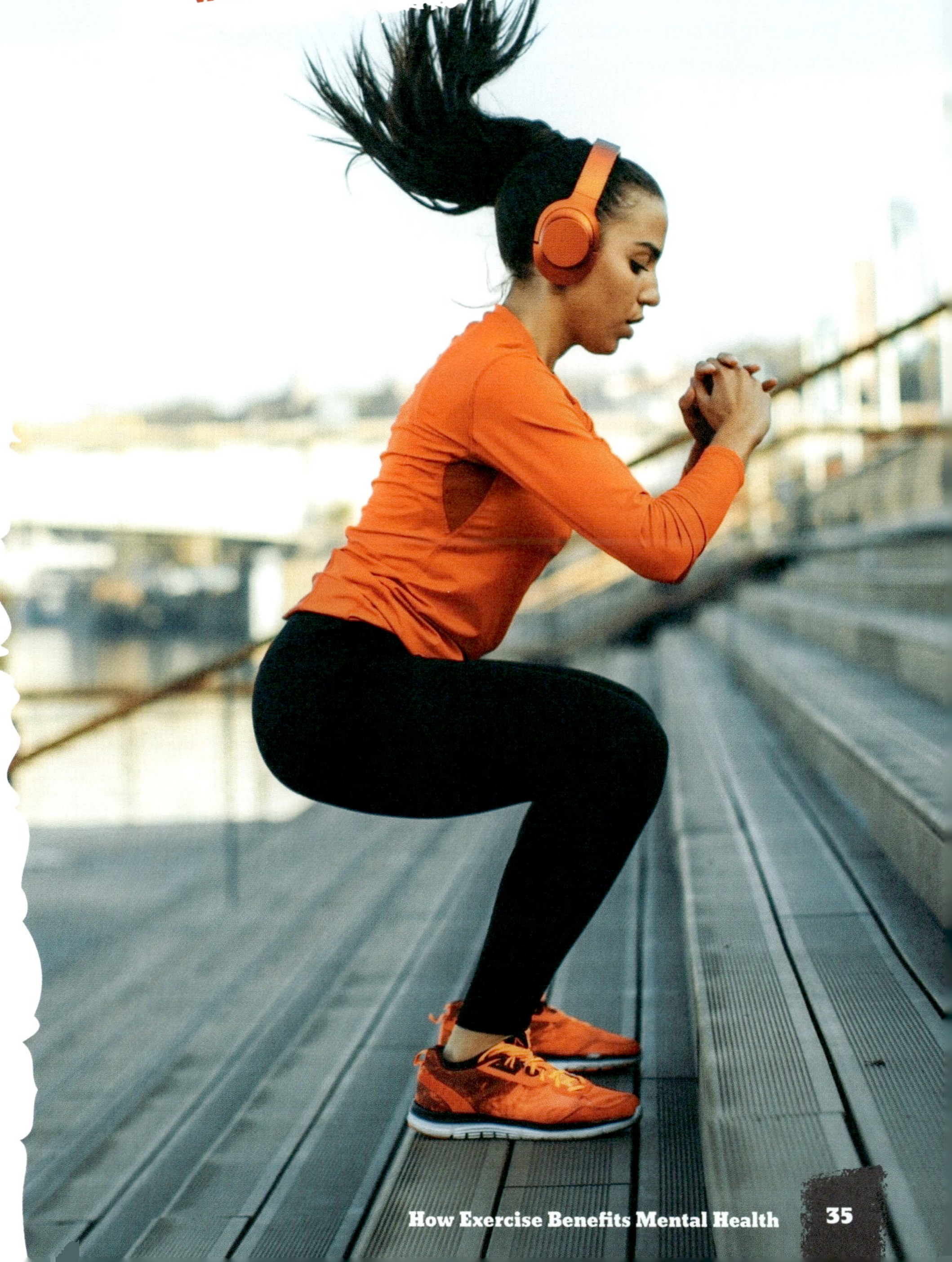

anxiety usually does in the first place, which is to fill your mind with an endless procession of worrisome thoughts.

While you are exercising, you are basically forced to focus your attention on the exercise at hand. Whether you are lifting a weight, jumping rope, or jogging on the track, you are automatically going to focus most of your attention on that task (for obvious reasons). This provides a much-needed break from anxiety, as you get a chance to put those recurring thoughts to the side and direct your brain power elsewhere!

THE SILENT KILLER

While we have always assumed that being stressed out all the time was obviously damaging to our health, the magnitude of this damage has become much more understood in recent times. Stress has been linked to so many illnesses and health conditions that it has come to be known as the "silent killer." With a name that intimidating, the need to cut out any unnecessary stress from your daily life is obviously a priority!

Clinical Nursing Research, a peer-reviewed publication dealing with an array of healthcare issues and interventions, published a study that pulled together the results of 19 different studies that all sought to examine the relationship between increased exercise and reduced anxiety in more than 3,000 test subjects. Researchers found that every one of these subjects showed a significant reduction in anxiety levels brought about by increased physical activity. Furthermore, the results seemed to be better among individuals only implementing increased exercise as opposed to those combining more exercise with other behavioral interventions.

EXERCISE AND STRESS

Due to the ridiculously fast pace of the world we live in today, people are stressed out more than ever before. You are probably no stranger to this feeling. Each day, there seems to be an endless number of

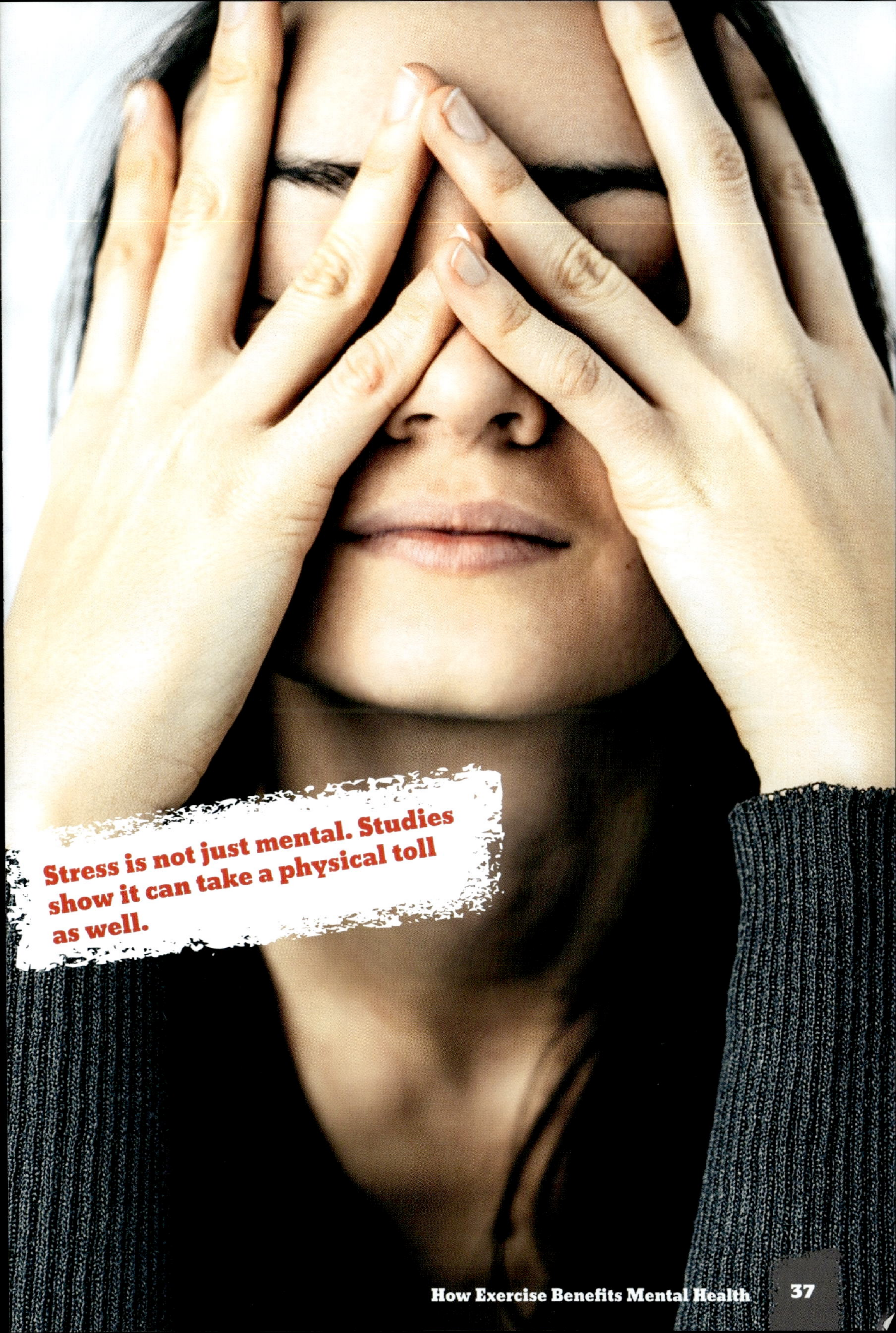

Stress is not just mental. Studies show it can take a physical toll as well.

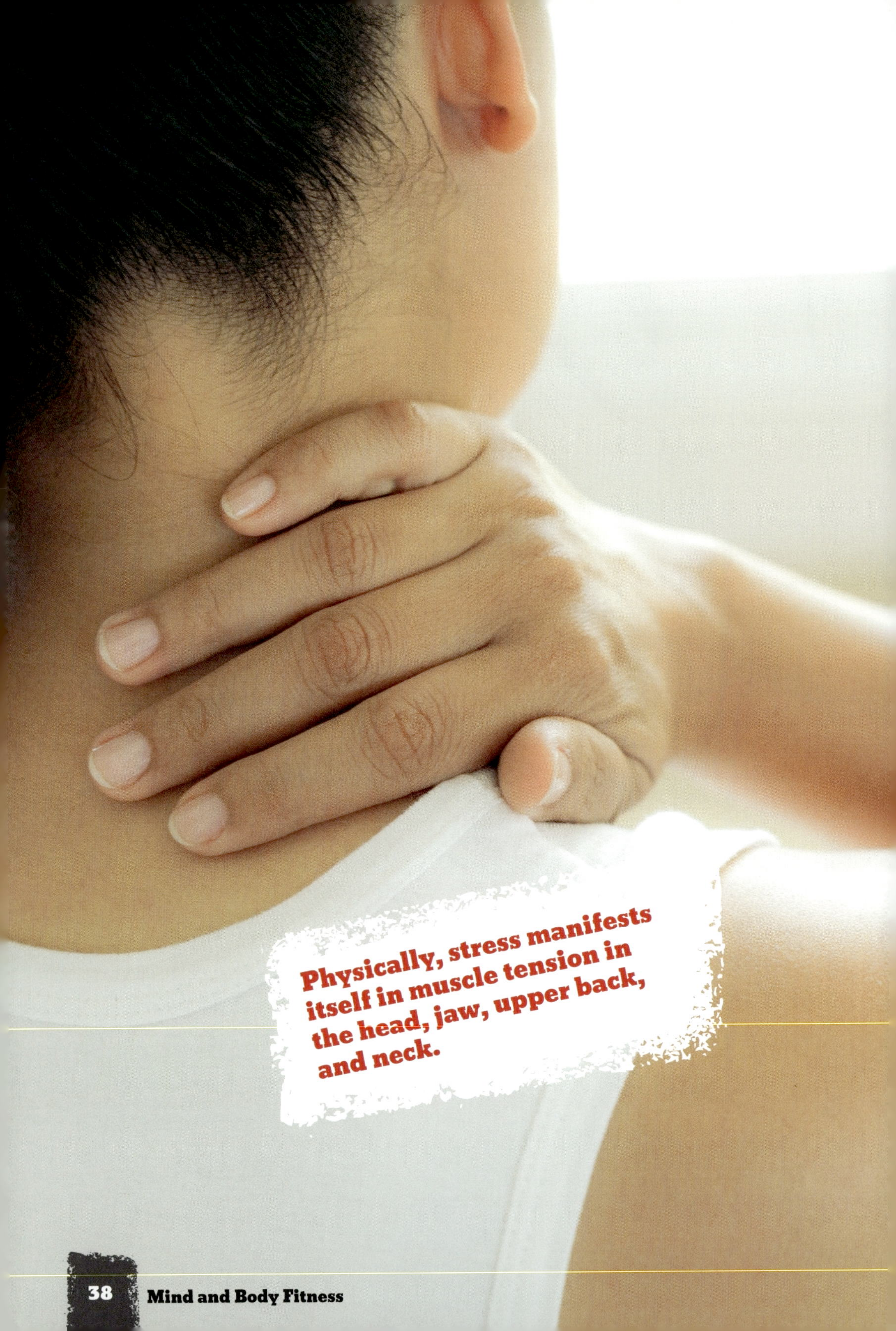

Physically, stress manifests itself in muscle tension in the head, jaw, upper back, and neck.

to-do's and responsibilities demanding your attention. While it is impossible to completely eliminate stress from your life, getting rid of the excess is imperative. Stress elicits an essential response from our bodies that was designed to help us deal with sudden life-threatening situations. This emotion is not something that was instilled in human beings to be felt all the time, as many people today are experiencing. In fact, chronic stress has been linked to a wide range of very serious health problems. Unrelenting stress is proven to cause everything from heart disease, obesity, and even premature death.

Fortunately, exercise is once again here for you when it comes to dealing with stress. The **endogenous** hormones released during exercise, which we have discussed several times, play a role in improving your mood, but many of the physical symptoms of stress can also be mitigated through exercise. As you have probably noticed during really stressful periods, certain muscle groups in your body seem to become increasingly tight and filled with tension. This is largely due to a subconscious reaction to stress that causes you to tense up and clench particular muscles. For most of us, this becomes noticeable in the head, jaw, and upper back. The constant contraction of these muscles causes **muscle adhesions** that limit your ability to move without pain and discomfort. Through exercise, these areas are able to contract and relax as they were intended to.

The *Archives of Medical Science* describes in a study how exercise is great at stimulating certain reward pathways in the brain that effectively reduce stress levels. Researchers involved in this study explain how our bodies perceive exercise as a pleasurable experience on a hormonal level, and that this perception causes an increase in various chemicals in the body, such as dopamine and nitrous oxide, that allow the brain to more effectively deal with chronic stress.

This video provides even more support to the idea that exercise is a fantastic intervention in relieving some of the most prevalent mental health issues we face today.

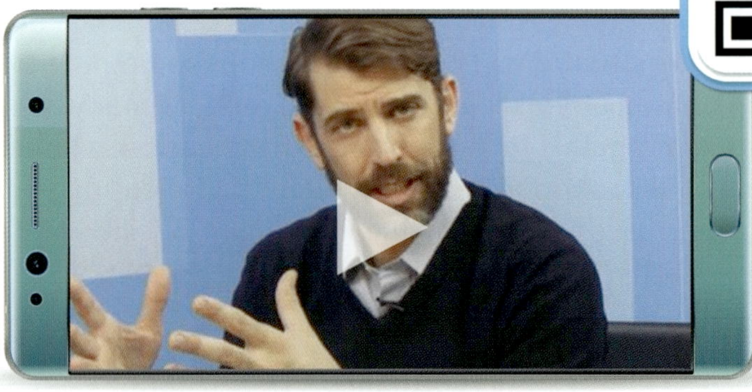

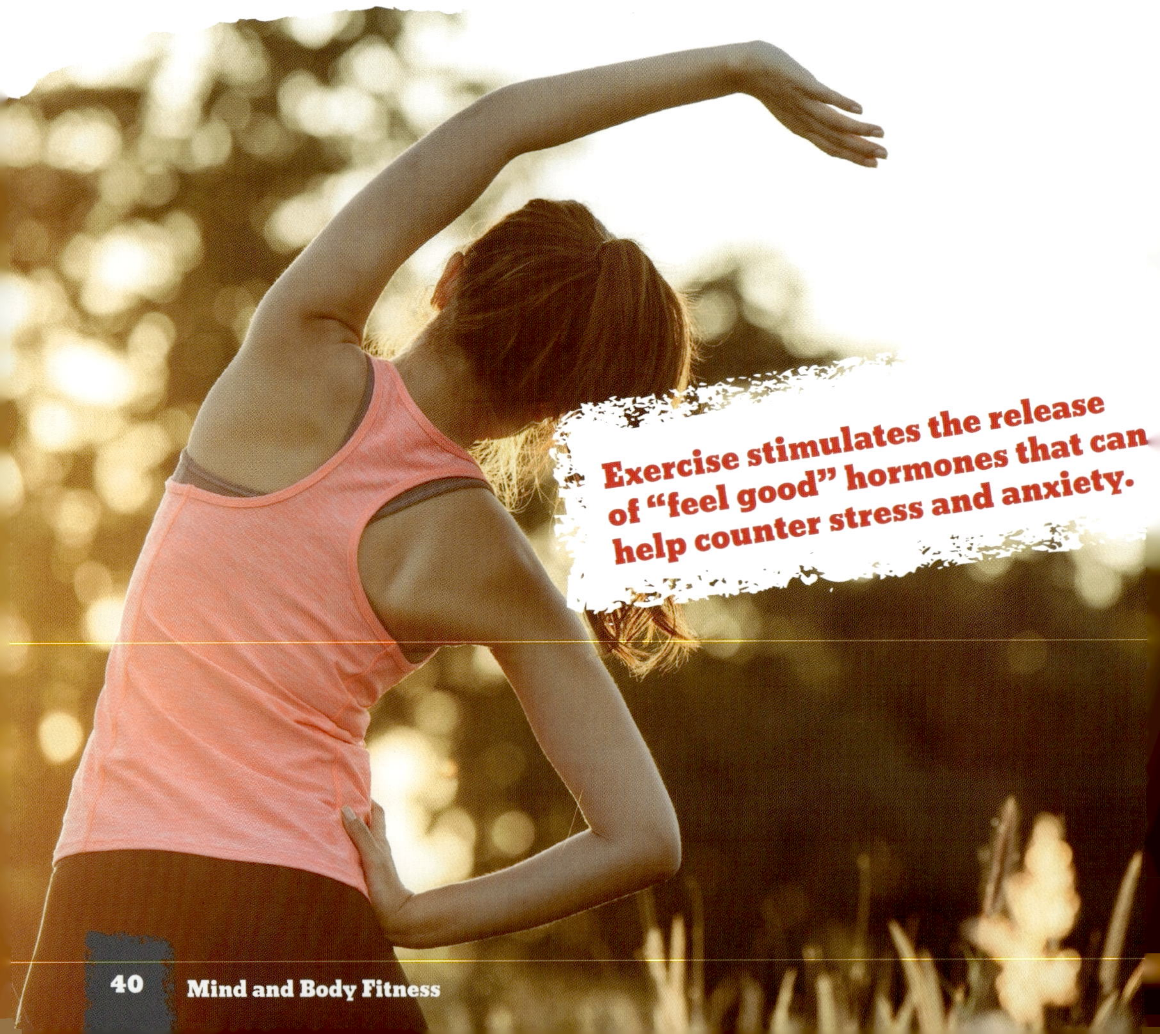

Exercise stimulates the release of "feel good" hormones that can help counter stress and anxiety.

COPING WITH ISOLATION

In the spring of 2020, most Americans and millions of people around the world were forced into quarantine due to the outbreak of a global pandemic. A novel coronavirus spread across the planet, infecting millions and killing hundreds of thousands. It was a dark time, and for many it was even more difficult due to the lack of social interaction and the loneliness of confinement.

For those in northern states, the timing was particularly bad as the order to shelter in place came just as seasonal depression was beginning to lift following a long winter. In this situation, people may find themselves in danger of entering a depression spiral, but that does not have to be the case. In situations of isolation, deepening depression is not an inevitable outcome.

People need to be aware, however, that it is possible for isolation to lead to or worsen depression. Data from the National Institutes of Health's PubMed Central database supports the existence of this link.

One thing that has been shown to help keep days from blurring together is to follow a routine. Routines help to define segments of the day and to provide things to look forward to doing each day.

Secondly, being alone doesn't mean you have to be alone. Get out of the house by going for a run or walk, or head to a park to read or to just people watch. Sunshine is an antidote for depression, as the vitamin D it provides is proven to help lift people's spirits.

A third remedy is to adopt a hobby. Perhaps it is something rekindled from the past, or just an interest yet to be tackled. Either way, activities like painting, crafting, and gardening can be effective in improving mental health.

Despite advancements in communication technology such as video chat, isolation can still become too much to bear for some. People that need to reach out for help should not feel badly about needing to do so. There are several virtual or remote options that offer professional therapy services. Therapists now offer sessions via video chat, or there are even apps like Calm and Headspace that focus on teaching appropriate coping mechanisms.

Whichever methods are employed, the important thing to remember is to keep trying. Depression is not predestined.

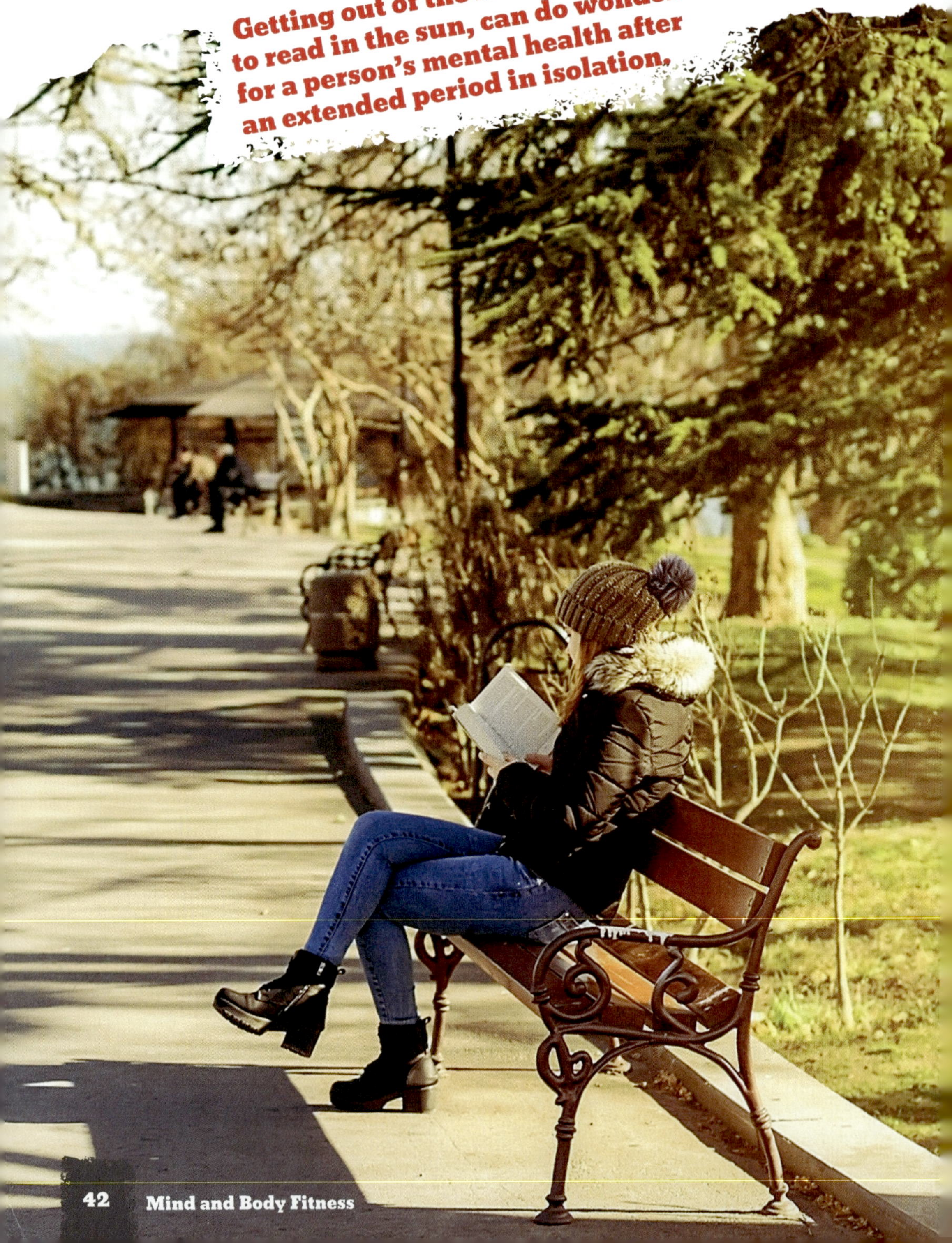

Getting out of the house, even if just to read in the sun, can do wonders for a person's mental health after an extended period in isolation.

Watch this to learn how to deal with anxiety and maintain good mental health in isolation.

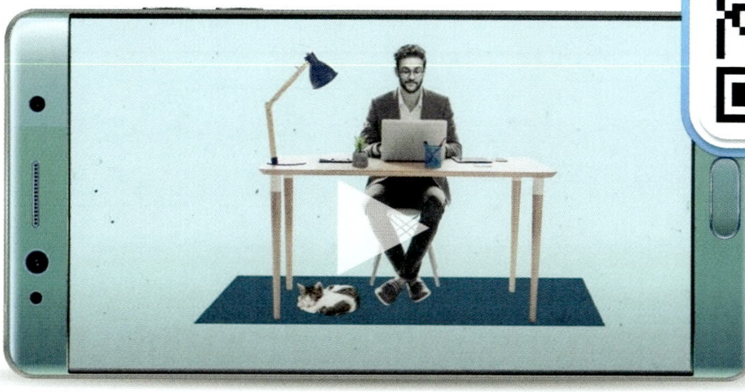

TEXT-DEPENDENT QUESTIONS

1. How does exercise directly affect the brain in a way that reduces many symptoms of depression?
2. Describe the term neurogenesis as it is used in this chapter describing how exercise alters neural pathways related to stress and anxiety.
3. What are two hormones mentioned in this chapter that are increased during exercise and that promote a reduction of depression, anxiety, and stress?

RESEARCH PROJECT

Mental health can be greatly improved through exercise due to hormonal responses, such as an increase in serotonin and dopamine. Dig a bit deeper into how these hormones interact with the brain. Find out exactly where these two hormones are produced in the body and what locations in the brain they travel to so they can positively affect our mood.

WORDS TO UNDERSTAND

cortisol—a glucocorticoid ($C_{21}H_{30}O_5$) produced by the adrenal cortex upon stimulation by ACTH that mediates various metabolic processes (such as gluconeogenesis), has anti-inflammatory and immunosuppressive properties, and whose levels in the blood may become elevated in response to physical or psychological stress

mind-body exercise—a form of exercise that combines body movement, mental focus, and controlled breathing to improve strength, balance, flexibility, and overall health

parasympathetic nervous system—the components of the central nervous system responsible for relaxation, digestion, and decreasing heart rate

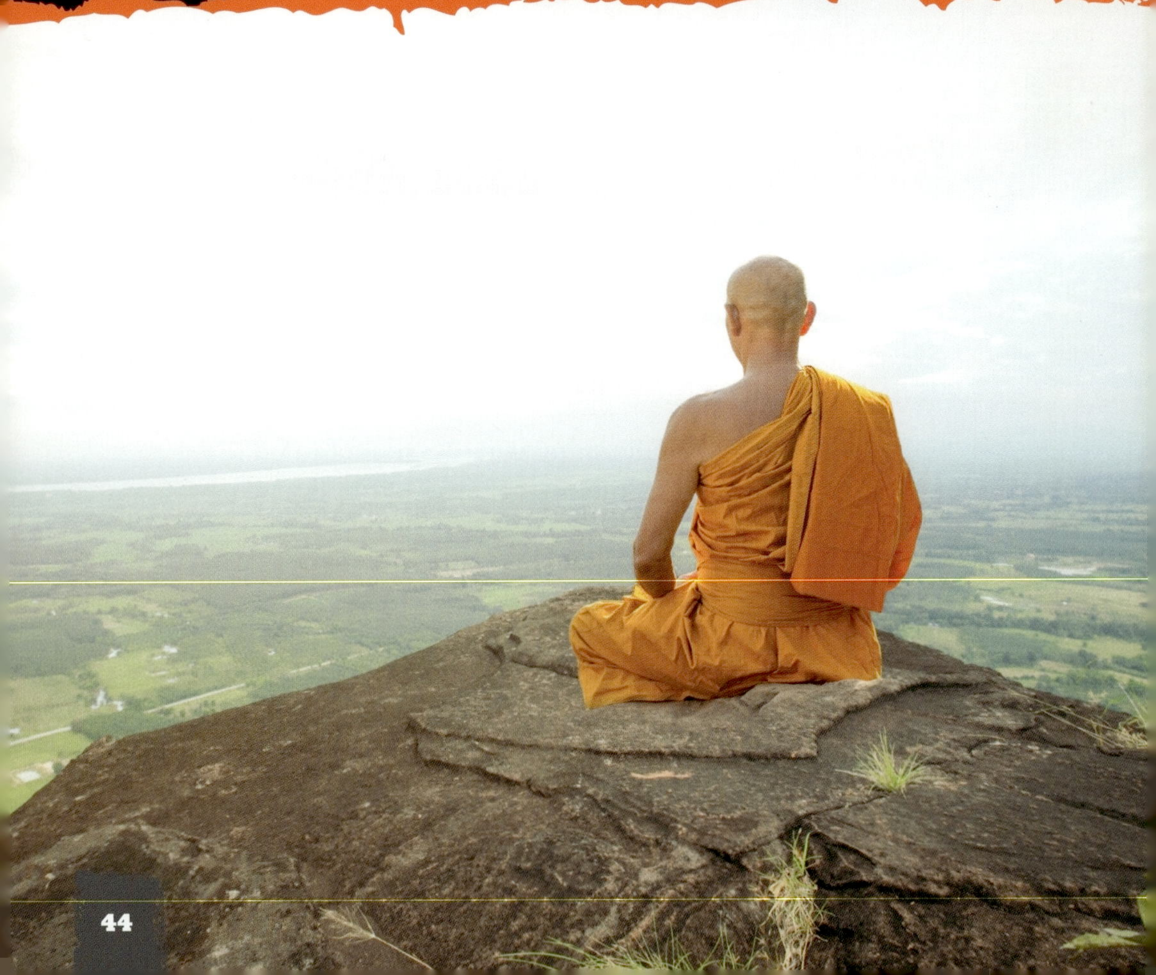

CHAPTER 4
MENTAL AND PHYSICAL BENEFITS OF YOGA

For most people, yoga is probably not the first thing that comes to mind pertaining to working out. Many of us have the idea that yoga is a gentle and soothing experience that mostly involves stretching. Given the huge amount of variation found within the practice of yoga, this is probably being done somewhere. However, yoga can be a fantastic way to push yourself physically while really getting into the mental side of fitness.

Although yoga is an ancient art form, it has found its way back into the mainstream in recent times. Ironically, this is largely due to the increased emphasis on physical fitness that we discussed in Chapter 1. More and more people are turning to yoga as a way to stay fit and limber, many of them doing so without even considering the mental aspect going on simultaneously.

There are several examples of research that support the claim that yoga is an effective **mind–body exercise**. Of the many variations of yoga, there are two in particular that, in their basic format, each challenge practitioners from both a mental and physical approach.

RESEARCH SUPPORTING THE GLOBAL BENEFITS OF YOGA

Many people are under the impression that yoga falls into the same category as simple meditation, being only a way to calm the mind and promote a sense of clarity and peace. While these are both true, the physical benefits available to those who practice yoga are also well documented.

In the *North American Journal of Medical Sciences,* one research article in particular provides a fantastic example of some of these physical benefits. In this example, a group of researchers synthesized the findings from numerous studies that were all conducted to observe the effects of yoga on various aspects of physical health. The studies that were analyzed focused on topics such as the nervous system, respiratory system, cardiovascular system, diabetes management, obesity, arthritis, cancer, and immune function. Additionally, each study came from a reputable, peer-reviewed source. The conclusions drawn from this insight into so many previous studies were interesting to say the least! In each of these studies, yoga was found to provide a significant benefit to the health condition related to the intervention. For example, yoga was shown as an effective way to reduce many of the common symptoms associated with asthma and chronic obstructive pulmonary disease. With regard to cardiovascular health, practicing yoga on a routine basis resulted in a significant reduction in blood pressure, heart rate, and even body mass index (BMI). Yoga was even shown to be an effective tool in reducing many of the symptoms brought about by arthritis. Although there is a large

BALANCING STRENGTH AND RANGE OF MOTION

For the majority of individuals who work out on a regular basis, the emphasis on flexibility and range of motion takes a back seat to other fitness goals. Most of us want to shed fat or add muscle to increase our strength and reach personal goals. While these are worthwhile pursuits, making sure you are still able to move efficiently and remain injury-free is also important. Yoga is a great addition to any fitness routine, as it provides a total body approach to lengthening muscles and connective tissue and making sure that you can actually use all that lean muscle to its fullest potential.

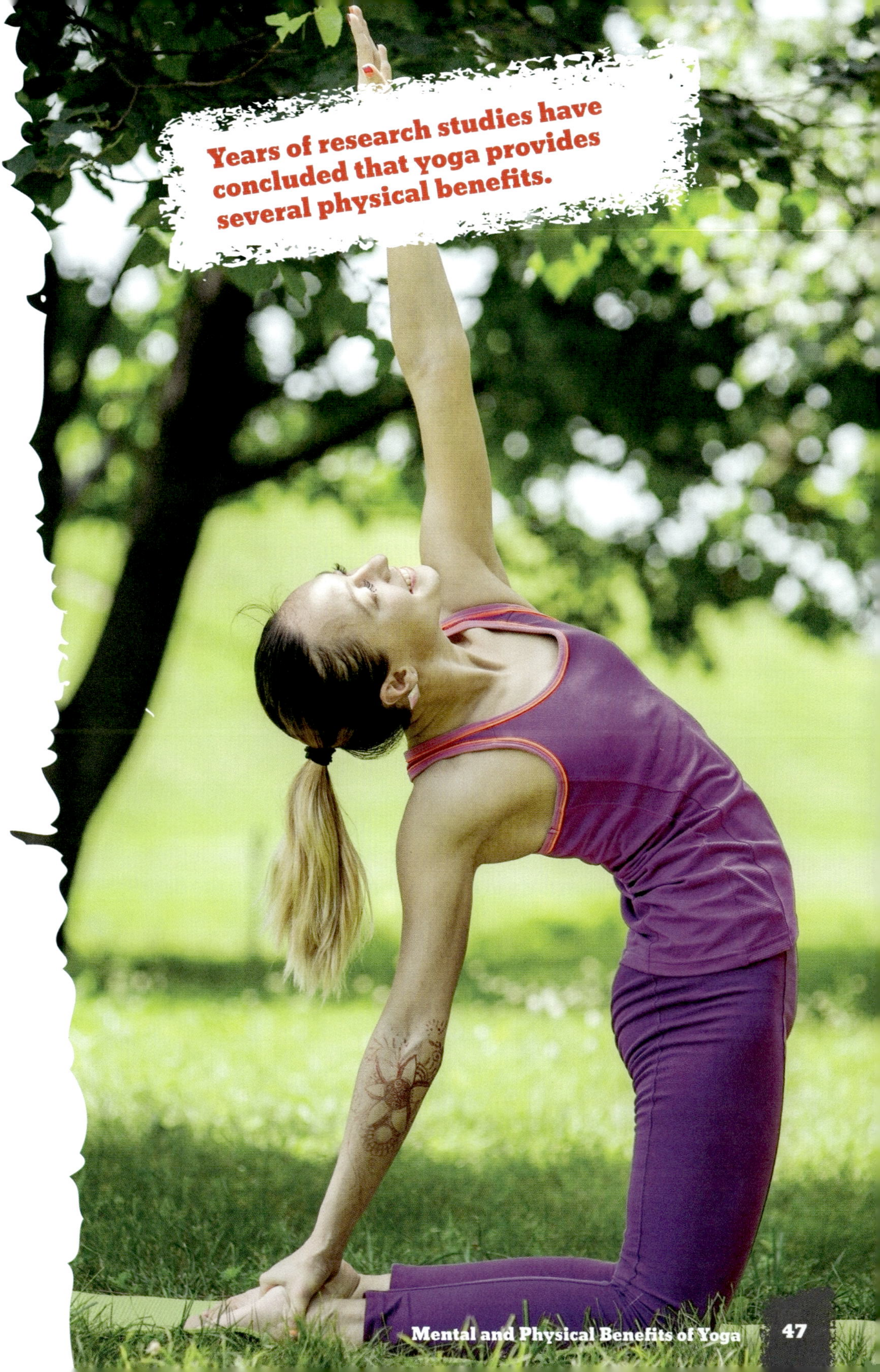

Years of research studies have concluded that yoga provides several physical benefits.

amount of research that supports practicing yoga to improve physical health, this article provided remarkable insight into just how numerous these physical benefits can be.

There is also a plethora of data available showing the mental benefits provided by practicing yoga. Even though this is probably not as surprising as the notion that yoga is great for physical fitness, it is still important to be aware of the reputable research available in support of this practice as a mental exercise as well. In *The International Journal of Yoga,* researchers observed the effects of one to two 90-minute yoga sessions per week for a period of one month across 25 subjects. To make the results of this study more applicable for the general population, subjects' age ranged from twenty to seventy-five years. The main variables tested were chronic stress and anxiety. While anxiety levels were recorded using basic outcome measures (standardized questionnaires), stress was observed by measuring the level of salivary amylase in each subject before and after the intervention. Salivary amylase is a chemical produced in the body during periods of heightened stress, when the **parasympathetic nervous system** is inactive and unable to mitigate the biological changes that take place during stressful situations, such as an increase in **cortisol**, a stress hormone. At the conclusion of this study, results showed favorable outcomes for the subjects involved, even in spite of the large differences in age across the individuals. The scores observed on anxiety outcome measures were significantly lower post-testing than when measured before the intervention. Similarly, researchers observed a definite decrease in salivary amylase in each of the subjects than the data recorded pre-testing.

AN EXERCISE FOR MIND AND BODY

There is a variation of yoga out there for everyone ranging from those that challenge the body to those that strengthen the mind. The two forms described below are intended to provide an example of both ends of the spectrum.

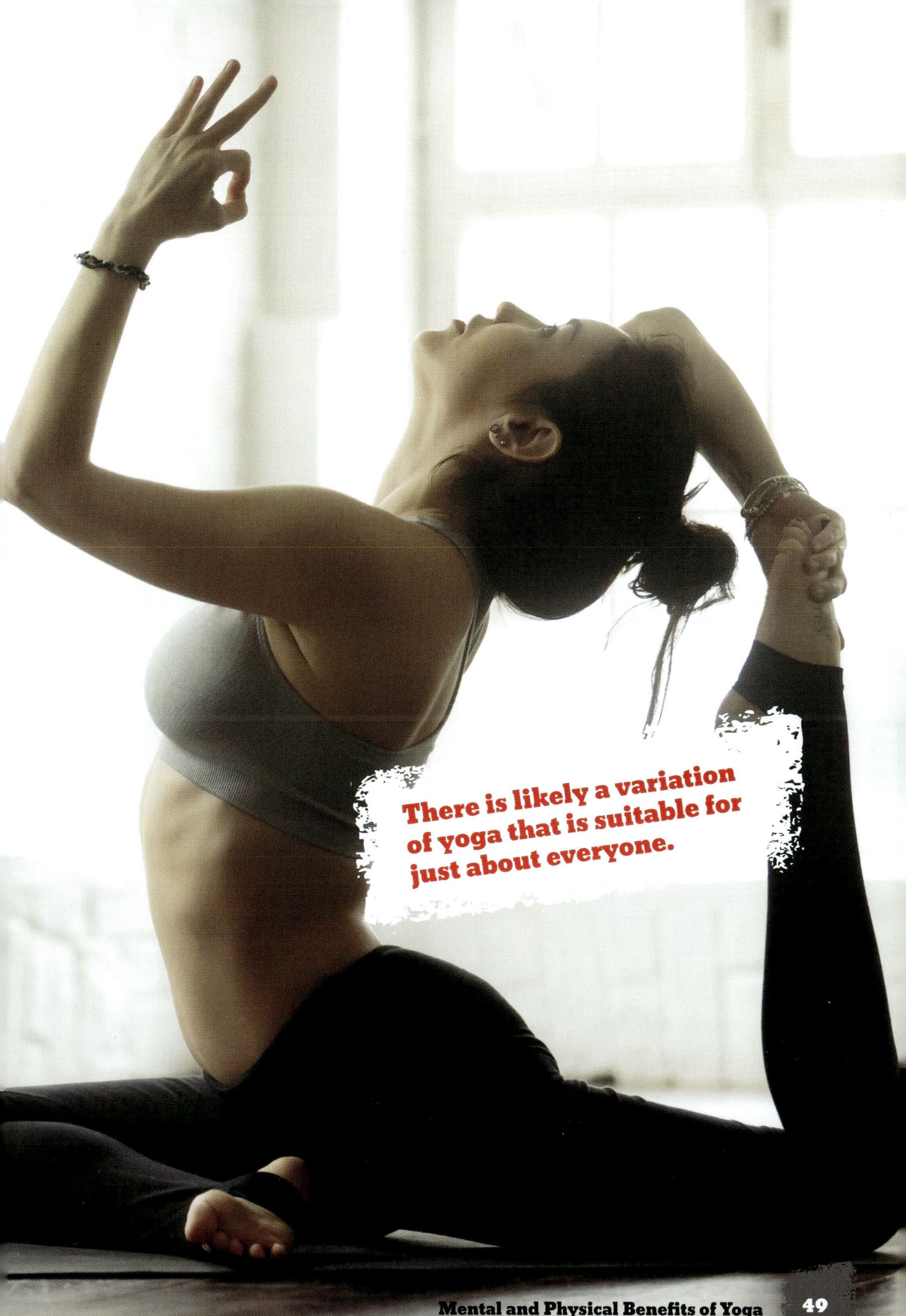

There is likely a variation of yoga that is suitable for just about everyone.

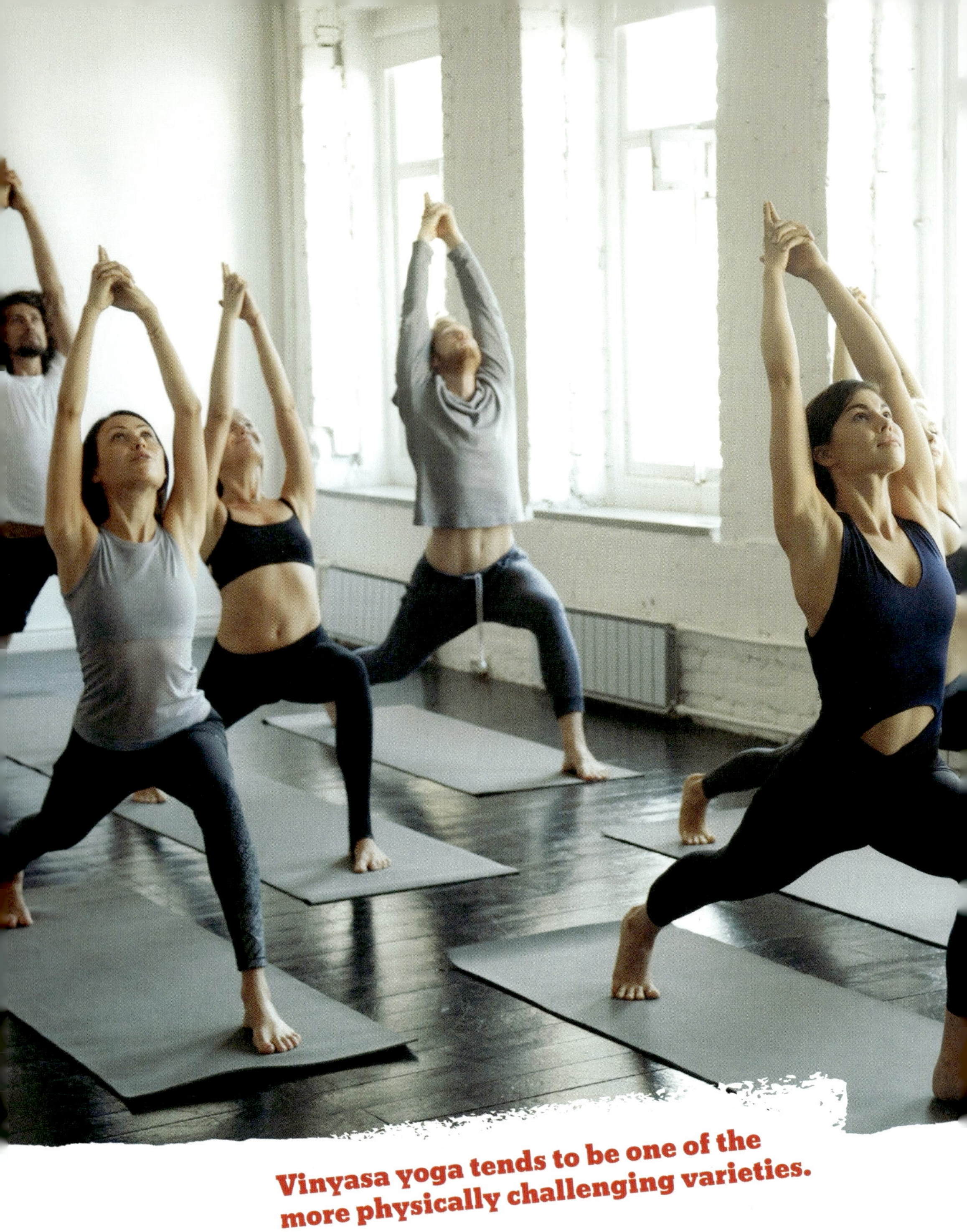

Vinyasa yoga tends to be one of the more physically challenging varieties.

Vinyasa Yoga

If you were to create a so-called "spectrum" of yoga with one end being the peaceful monk on a mountaintop and the other being an all-out physical challenge, Vinyasa yoga would certainly lean toward the latter end of this scale. This variation of yoga is characterized as a high-intensity approach that involves transitioning rather quickly through various poses. Unlike other forms of yoga, no two sessions involve the same poses or sequence of movements. Breathing remains an important aspect of Vinyasa, as the breath is one of the key components of yoga in general. Transitioning the body from one pose to the next is accomplished by "breathing" into the next position. Even though the fast-paced nature of Vinyasa yoga is physically challenging, being able to control the rate of breathing during sometimes difficult movement transitions is very important.

YOGA WITH AN ATTITUDE

Vinyasa yoga is basically everything that those unfamiliar with yoga think it is not. While you will certainly still improve your mind and body connection during each session, the experience will be anything but sitting cross-legged with your eyes closed in complete peace. Vinyasa is a shining example of how there are enough variations of yoga to suit anyone and everyone willing to vary their exercise routine.

Vinyasa yoga is an extremely effective way to simultaneously improve your mental and physical fitness. Even though the physical challenge involved with this technique is readily apparent, being in tune with the flow of your breathing adds a mental component in the process. Vinyasa forces you to manage the physical sensations from your body while still keeping your focus on your inward state of mind at the same time.

Here are a couple of videos that illustrate the overall format and approach behind the first yoga variation discussed in this chapter: Vinyasa.

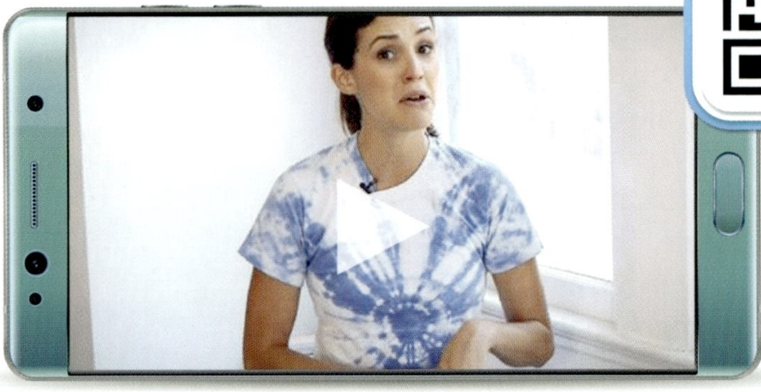

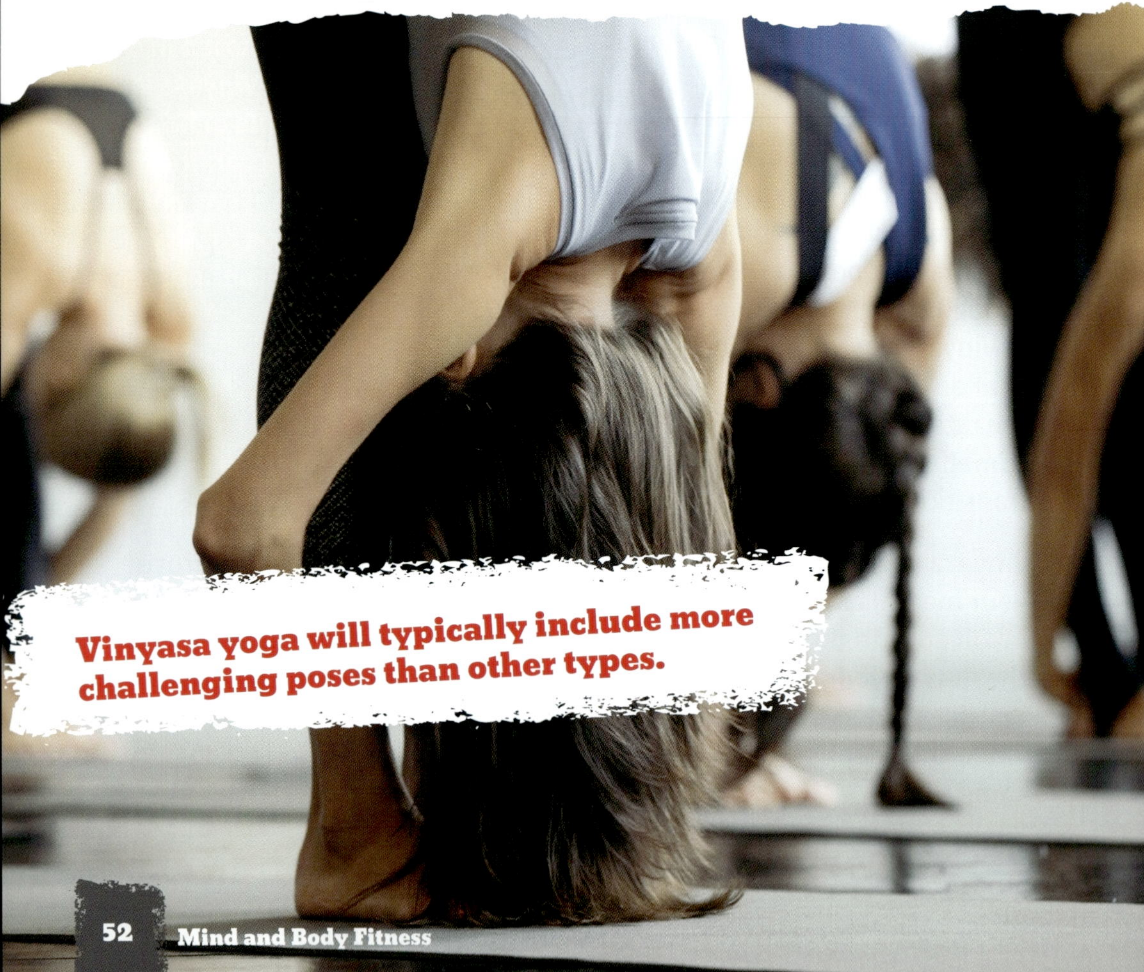

Vinyasa yoga will typically include more challenging poses than other types.

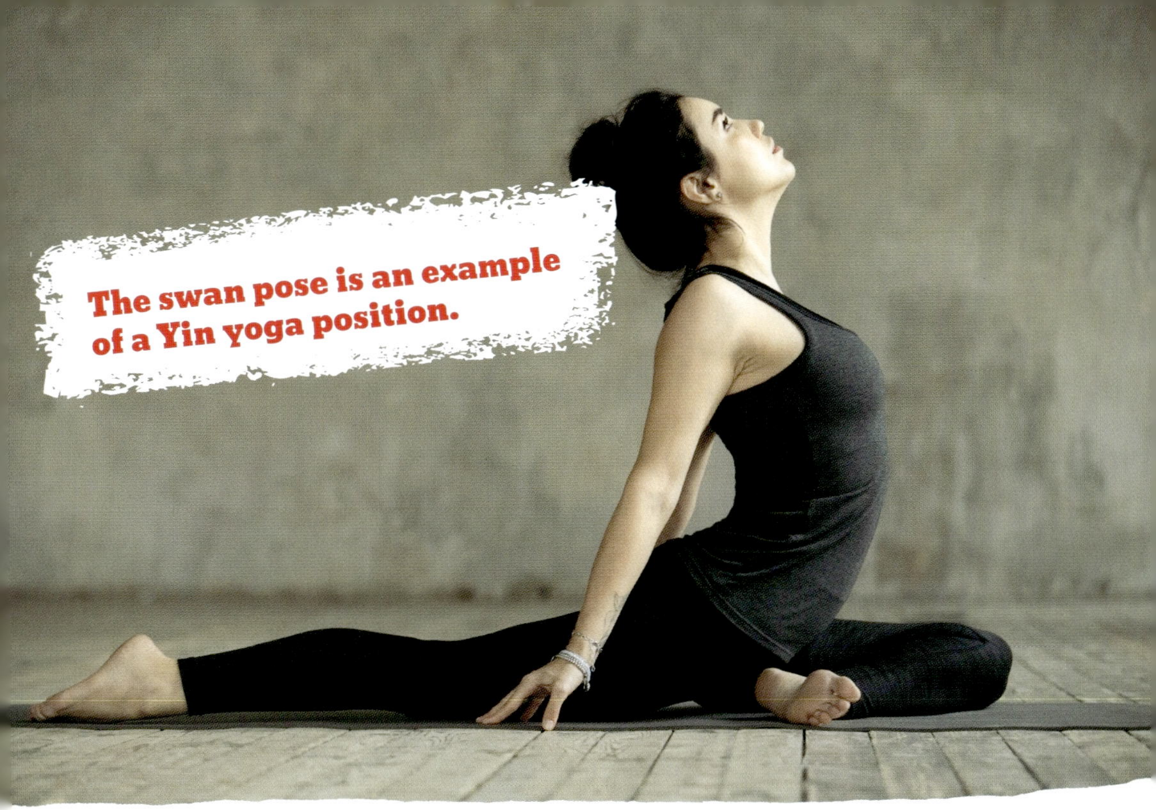

The swan pose is an example of a Yin yoga position.

Yin Yoga

On the other end of this hypothetical spectrum, we have Yin yoga. This variation more accurately fits the common perception of yoga in mainstream society, but there is very much a physical aspect to the technique.

The primary focus of Yin yoga is to stretch and lengthen the connective tissue throughout your body. A typical session involves 20 poses that are held for a considerable length of time, sometimes up to five minutes. Due to the longer duration of each pose, muscle fibers and connective tissue that are normally tight and sensitive due to stress, resistance training, and poor posture are allowed to finally open up and release excess tension. The mental aspect of Yin yoga is also emphasized by holding certain positions for an extended period of time, as the quiet and serene environment implemented in the studio is favorable for focusing on breathing and making the effort to quiet your thoughts easier as you restore range of motion throughout the body. Many of the poses are particularly effective at stretching areas of the body prone to developing tension and stress, such as the lower back, hamstrings, and hip muscles.

If you are looking for a more traditional form of yoga that still provides a great way to improve your mental and physical fitness, Yin yoga may be the appropriate variation for you. If you have certain "problem" areas throughout your body that seem to constantly feel stiff and uncomfortable, this form of yoga has the potential to provide relief to these hotspots while also allowing you to focus on channeling your thought pattern into precisely processing the feedback from your musculature and restoring proper breathing.

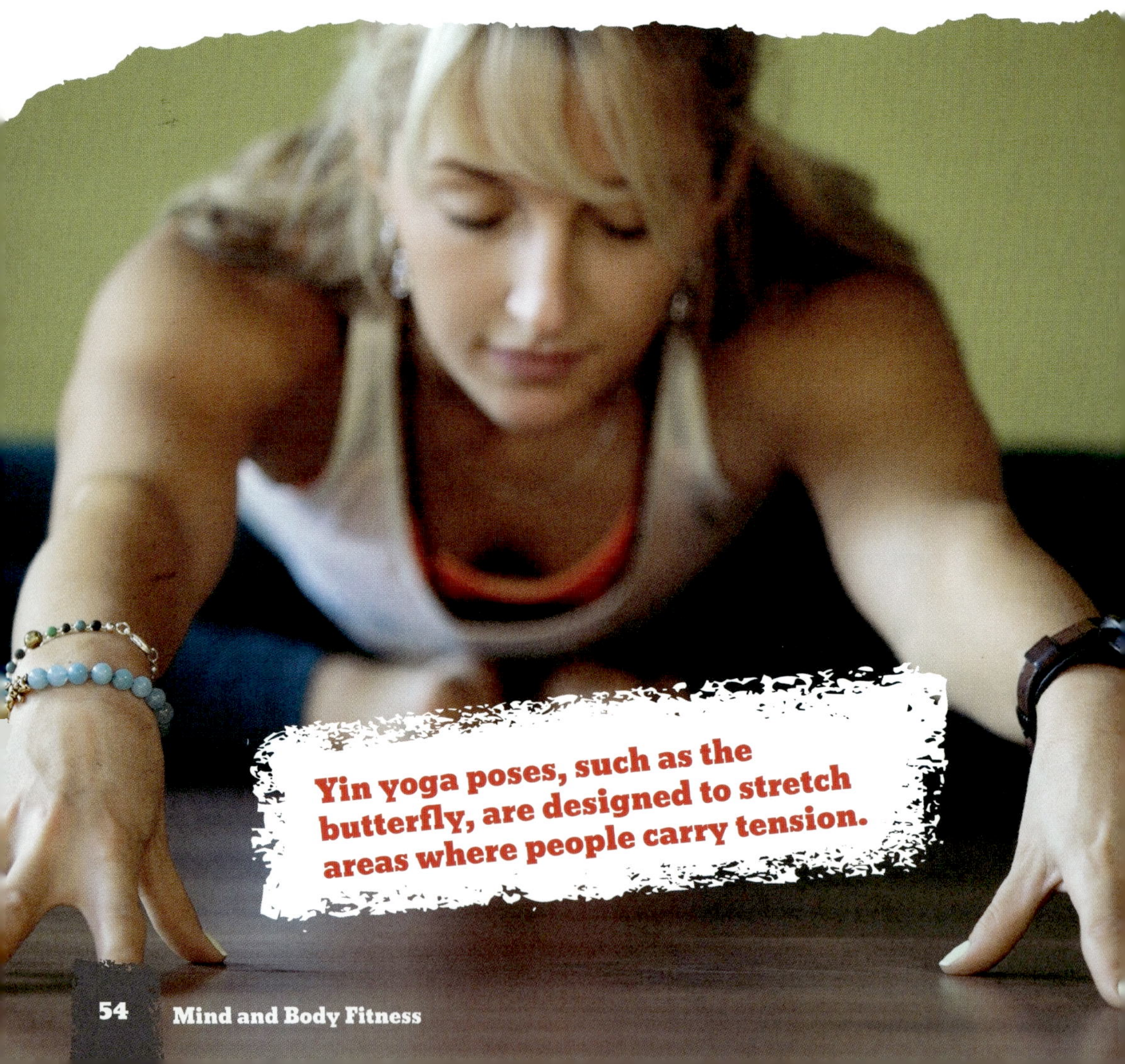

Yin yoga poses, such as the butterfly, are designed to stretch areas where people carry tension.

Here are a couple of videos that illustrate the overall format and approach behind the second yoga variation discussed in this chapter: Yin.

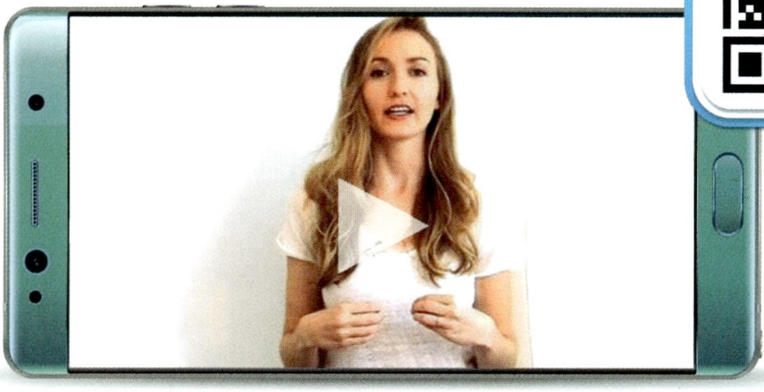

TEXT-DEPENDENT QUESTIONS

1. Describe two key differences between the Vinyasa and Yin forms of yoga as they are detailed in this chapter.
2. How many poses are included in a session of the Yin method of yoga?
3. While both forms of yoga detailed in this chapter provide mind and body benefits, which form would be considered more of a physical workout?

RESEARCH PROJECT

Although we only detailed two forms of yoga in this chapter, there is a vast array of methods out there, which is unsurprising when you consider just how ancient yoga actually is. Just about every variation of yoga is effective at providing some form of mental and physical benefits. Research to find another form of yoga besides the two mentioned in this chapter. Describe the basic format of the variation you choose and list the primary ways this specific yoga variation benefits fitness from a physical and mental perspective.

WORDS TO UNDERSTAND

Jing—a word often used when practicing Tai Chi that dictates mental quietness

Qi—the circulating life force whose existence and properties are the basis of much Chinese philosophy and medicine

Song—a Chinese word used in Tai Chi to symbolize relaxation

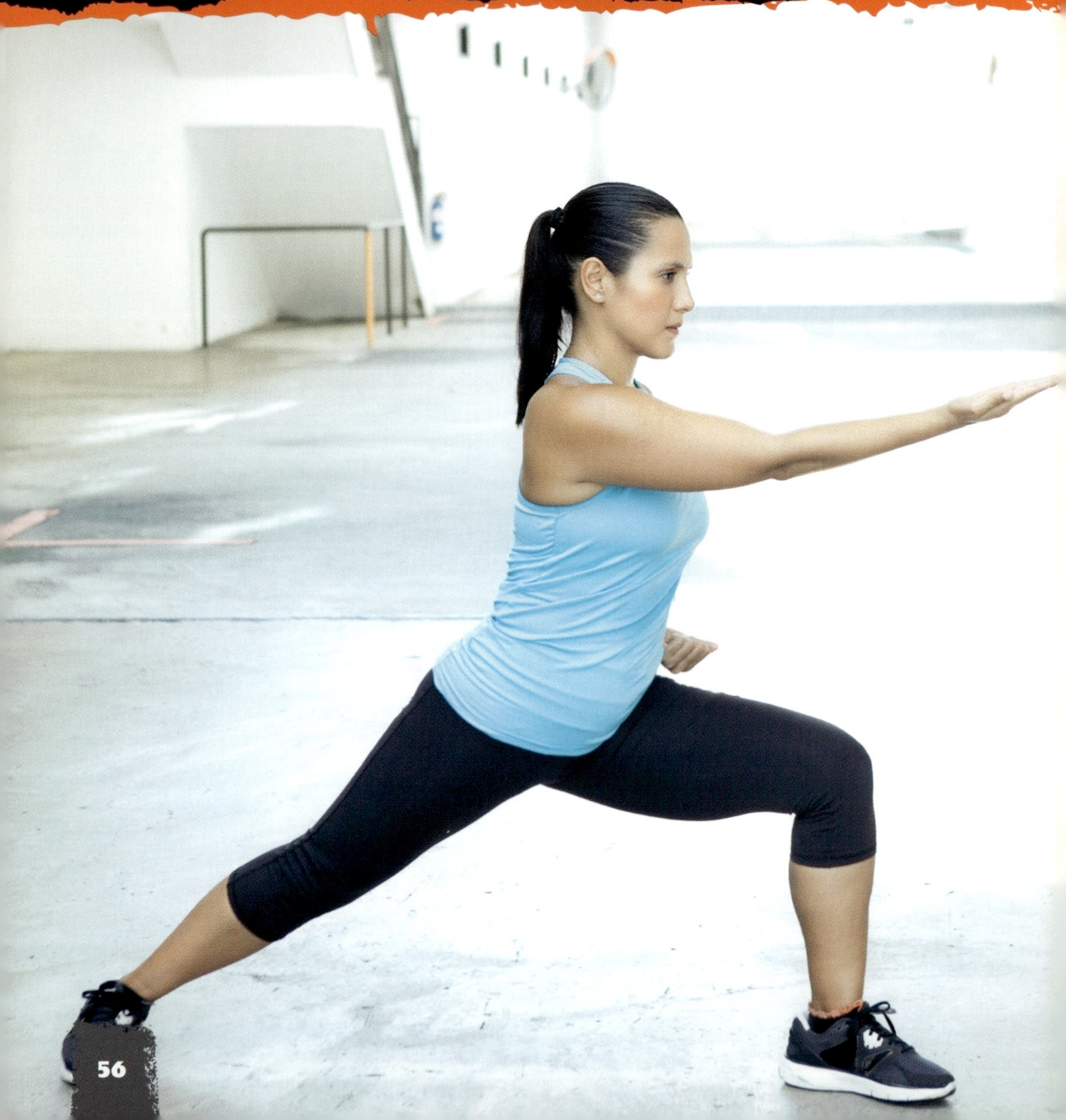

CHAPTER 5
TAI CHI: BALANCE THE MIND AND BODY

Tai Chi is another ancient form of exercise that seeks to unite the mind and body. This art, although it has a large number of variations, is similar to yoga in that precise, intentional movements are coupled with breath control and mental focus. Probably the easiest way to differentiate the two is the amount of time spent holding a particular pose. With yoga, even the more dynamic forms, there is always an emphasis placed on holding a pose for a certain period of time before moving on to the next. In Tai Chi, the entire technique is designed to flow through a series of movements with no prolonged stopping at any point. Another way to think about the difference between these two techniques is that during yoga, you are essentially stretching throughout the session as a way to relax. Tai Chi involves first entering a state of relaxation, or **Song**, so that your body is loose enough to be allowed to stretch.

With Tai Chi, the importance of improving your mental and physical fitness is emphasized as the foundation of the entire art seeks to unite the mind and body by harnessing what is known as **Qi**, or life energy, and allowing this energy to flow throughout the body. By controlling the breathing throughout this flow of movement, practitioners of Tai Chi are allowed to promote a state of **Jing**, which is very similar to entering a state of mindfulness.

Although it is not usually as intense as many forms of yoga, Tai Chi is still proven to be beneficial in both a mental and physical capacity. Following are examples of research supporting its use along with descriptions of several different variations of the method.

TAI CHI IN THE RESEARCH

It is fascinating that a form of exercise dating as far back as Tai Chi can still be supported even today through research as a beneficial practice for mind and body health. In a journal managed by the Psychiatric Clinics of North America, an article was published that described a meta-analysis carried out to provide insights into the efficacy of Tai Chi regarding improving mental health outcomes. Researchers were able to identify 21 randomized controlled trials and non-randomized comparison studies that concluded performing Tai Chi for up to an hour per day over the course of one year significantly increases psychosocial

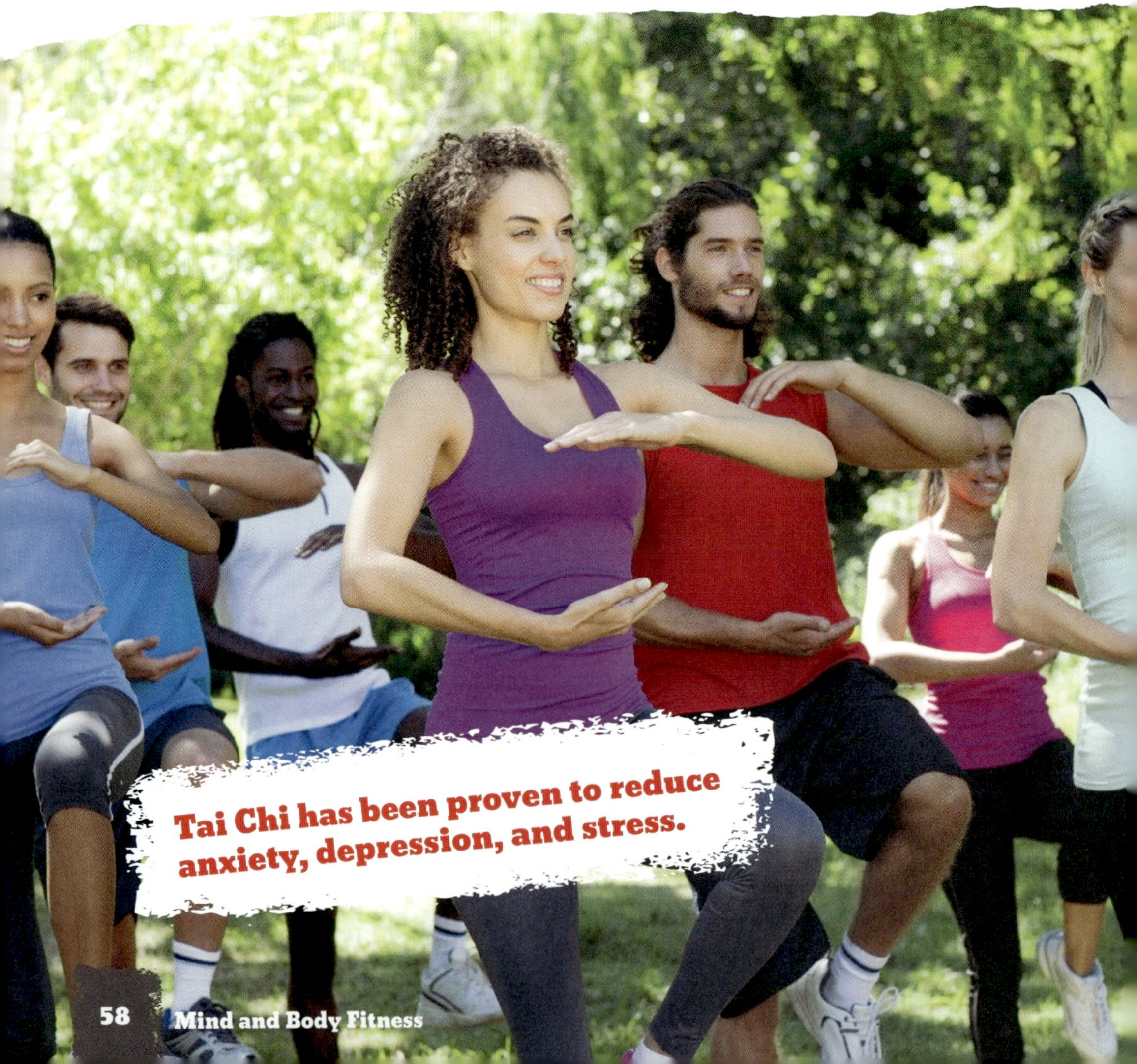

Tai Chi has been proven to reduce anxiety, depression, and stress.

well-being. This practice was also found to decrease stress, anxiety, and depression in community-dwelling individuals.

Another study published in the *International Journal of Behavioral Medicine* depicts a systemic review comprising of 42 studies that describe the effects of Tai Chi on mental health. The results of this review are very similar to the research above. Researchers concluded that, across various populations, Tai Chi is effective at reducing anxiety and depression as well as improving subjects' ability to manage stress.

VISITING THE ORIGINS OF TAI CHI

Tai Chi is a very old form of exercise that can be traced back to China. Most historians credit a monk named Zhang San Feng with creating this technique anywhere from 700 to 1,500 years ago. Interestingly enough, Tai Chi was originally created as a fighting art, much like karate or taekwondo. While Tai Chi has certainly experienced its share of variation over time, the basic concept of controlling the body and mind as one solitary unit has remained.

Research into Tai Chi goes much further than supporting its many benefits to mental health. In fact, an article included in the *Canadian Family Physician* journal states that over the past 45 years, there have been more than 500 trials and 20 systematic reviews published on the health benefits of Tai Chi. Among these studies, many focus specifically on general health and fitness. Researchers concluded that in this aspect alone, Tai Chi has been repeatedly supported as a means to improve balance and aerobic capacity, as well as increase force production in the lower limbs.

Since its creation, Tai Chi has been divided into five primary forms. While each of these variations differ in both their methodology and intent, the idea of combining the mind and body is universal.

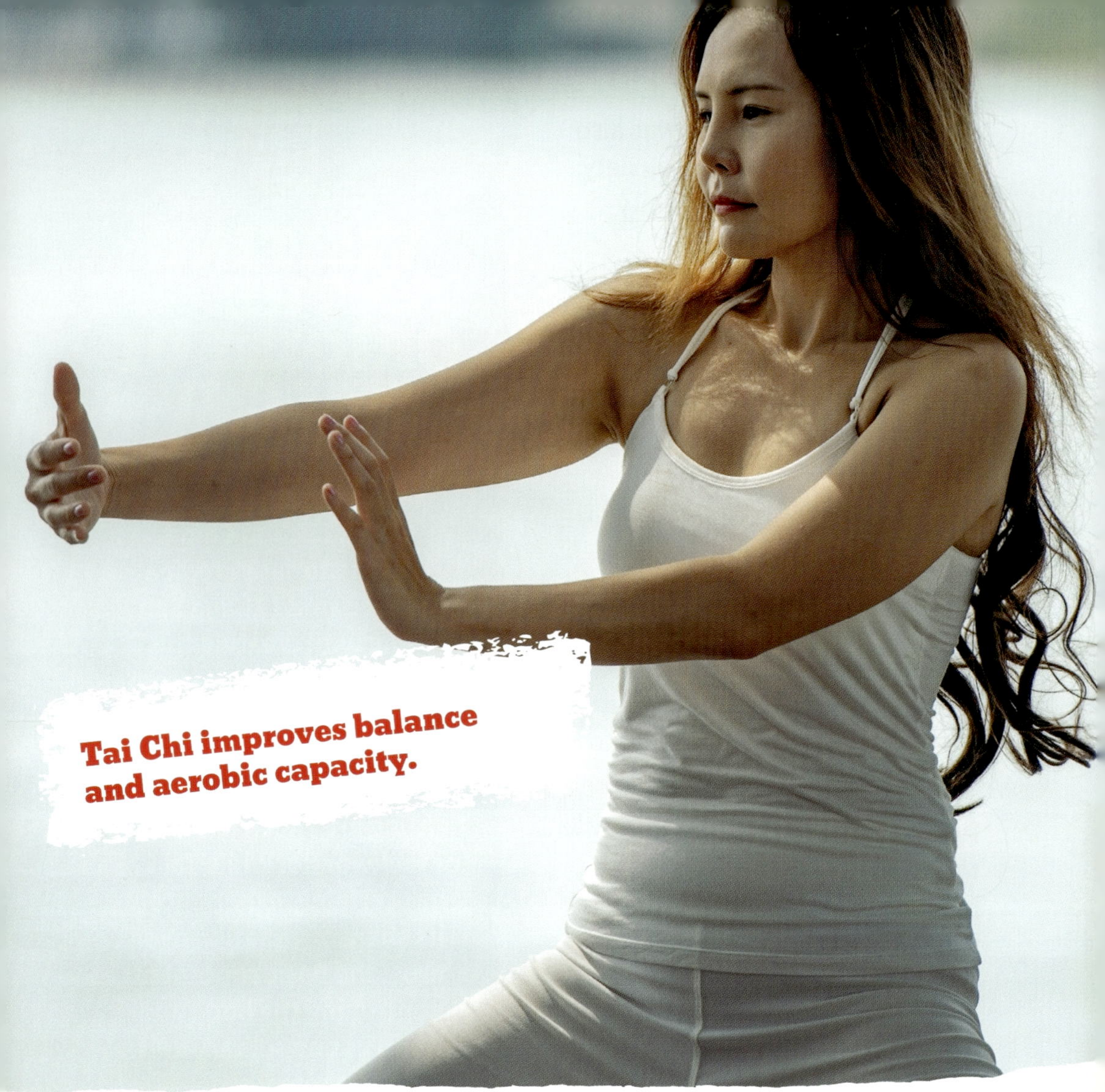

Tai Chi improves balance and aerobic capacity.

THE FIVE FORMS OF TAI CHI

Tai Chi owes much of its variation to several families that began practicing their own unique versions of what was originally considered a martial art. Although this art form was originally created by a monk as early as 1,500 years ago, it was this group of families that most likely brought Tai Chi into prominence.

Here is a brief video that provides some insight into the four most popular forms of Tai Chi.

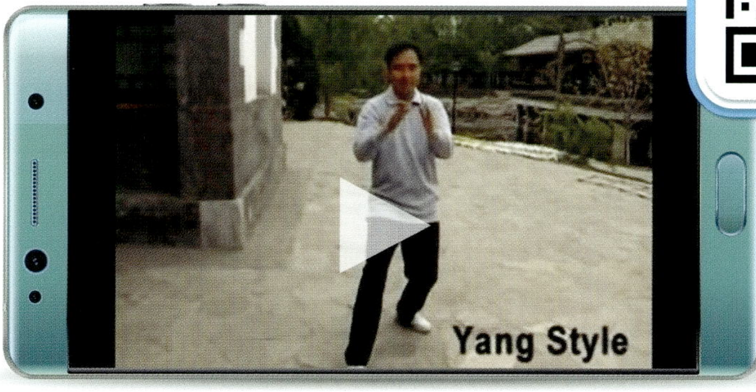
Yang Style

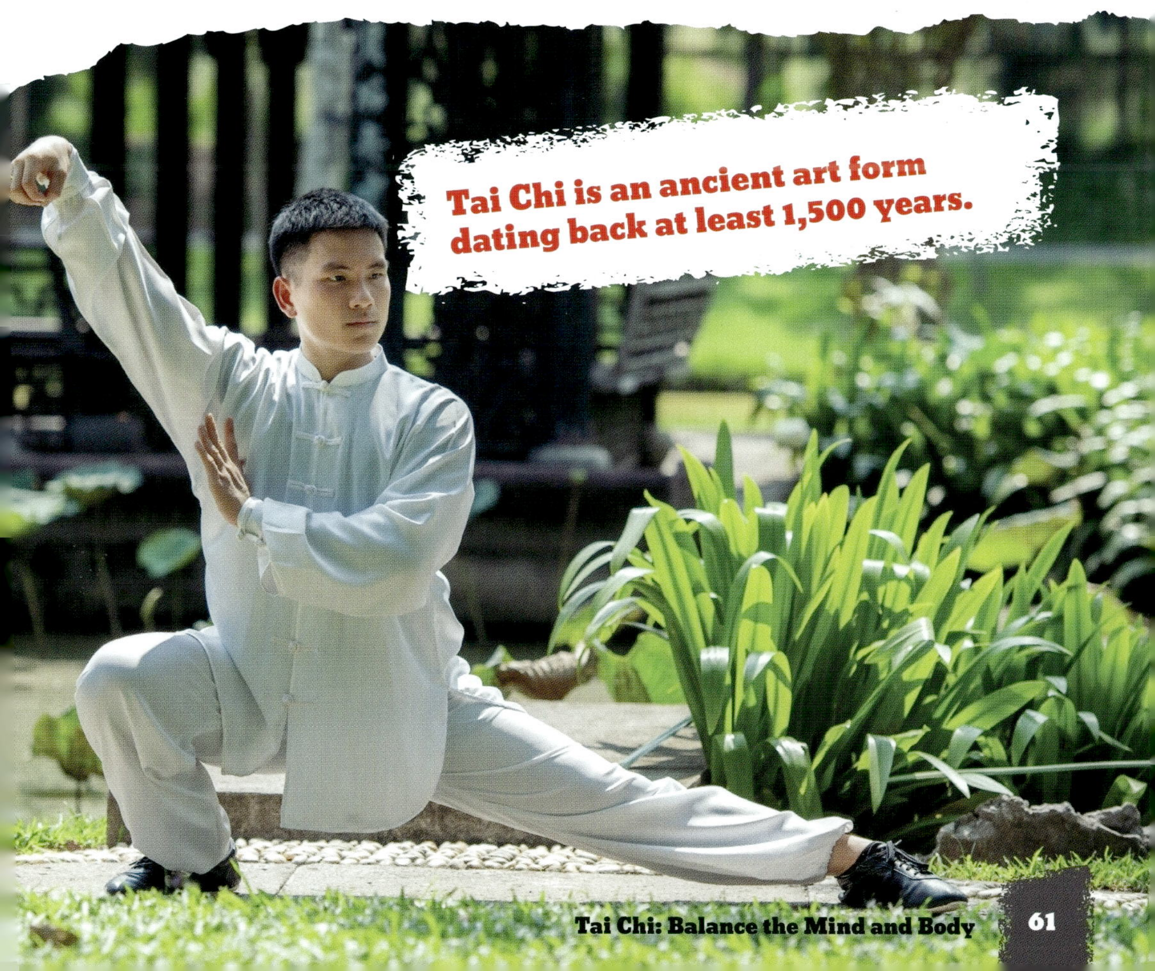
Tai Chi is an ancient art form dating back at least 1,500 years.

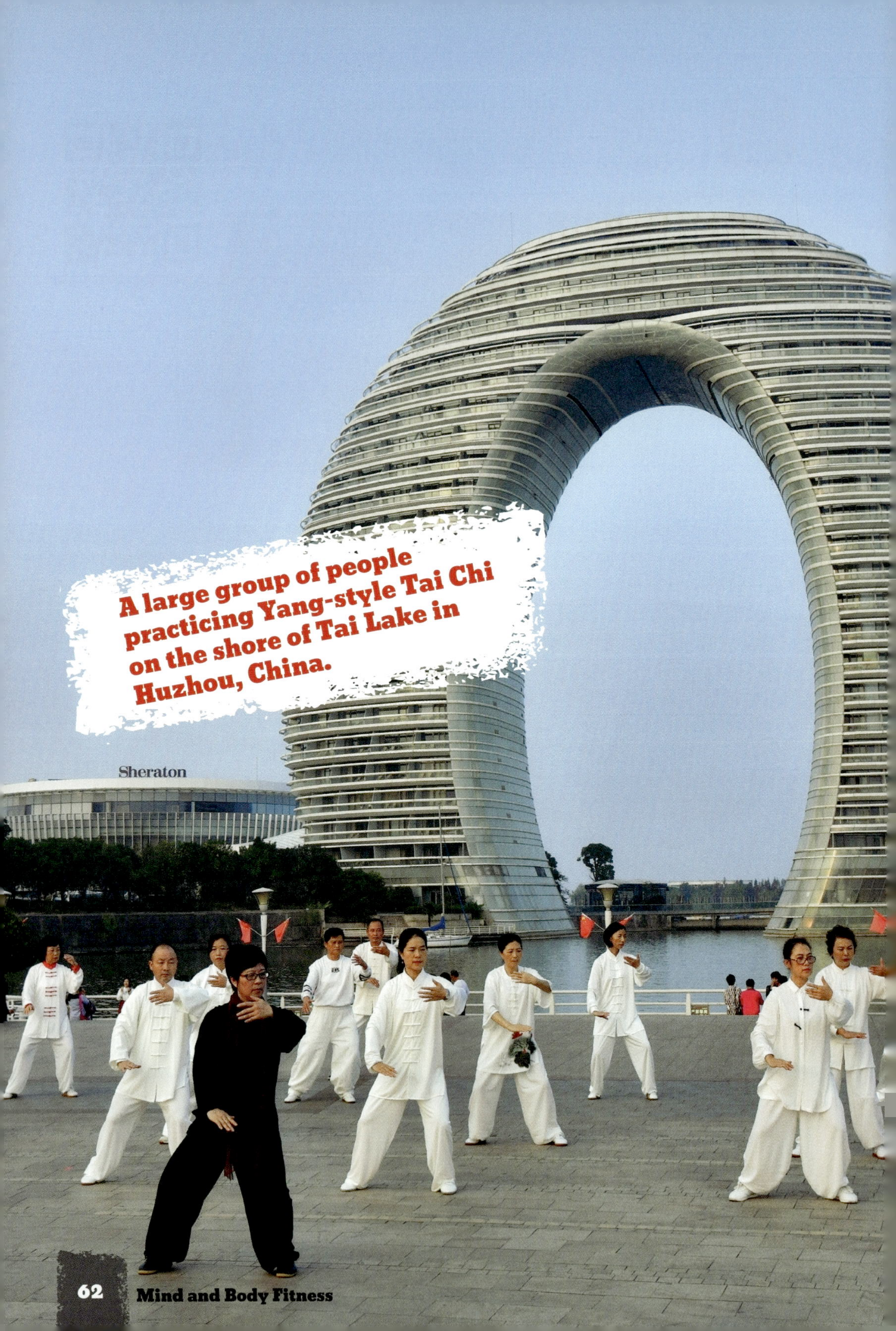

A large group of people practicing Yang-style Tai Chi on the shore of Tai Lake in Huzhou, China.

Chen Style

This version of Tai Chi is often considered the oldest variation. It is believed that the Chen family began practicing a unique form of the martial art around the seventeenth century. Due to this family adopting Tai Chi as a combat technique, the Chen style of Tai Chi incorporates more of a dynamic aspect than other variations.

Chen-style Tai Chi is made up of high-intensity movements such as kicking and striking, with the practitioner performing these movements from a crouched stance. Due to this stance, this form of Tai Chi is great at increasing leg strength and agility. While there are several slow and methodical movements included in this technique, these are quickly alternated with the fighter-like movements that make Chen style unique.

Yang Style

The Yang variation of Tai Chi is often considered the most popular version of the art. This family modified the Chen style in a way that emphasized less athleticism in favor of a more graceful, gentle form of movement. This form of Tai Chi was actually taught to the elite guards of the Imperial family.

Yang-style Tai Chi is great at improving flexibility and range of motion due to the large, full-body movements involved. The widespread utilization of this variation is due, in part, to its ability to be effectively practiced by individuals who may be older or not physically fit enough to perform more explosive movements.

Wu Style

This variation of Tai Chi is particularly effective at improving balance and controlling one's center of gravity. The Wu style of Tai Chi owes its inception to the Wu family, as one of its members was actually included in the group of Imperial guards instructed in the aforementioned Yang version.

Unlike other forms of Tai Chi that involve remaining centered throughout the routine, this version places an emphasis on moving

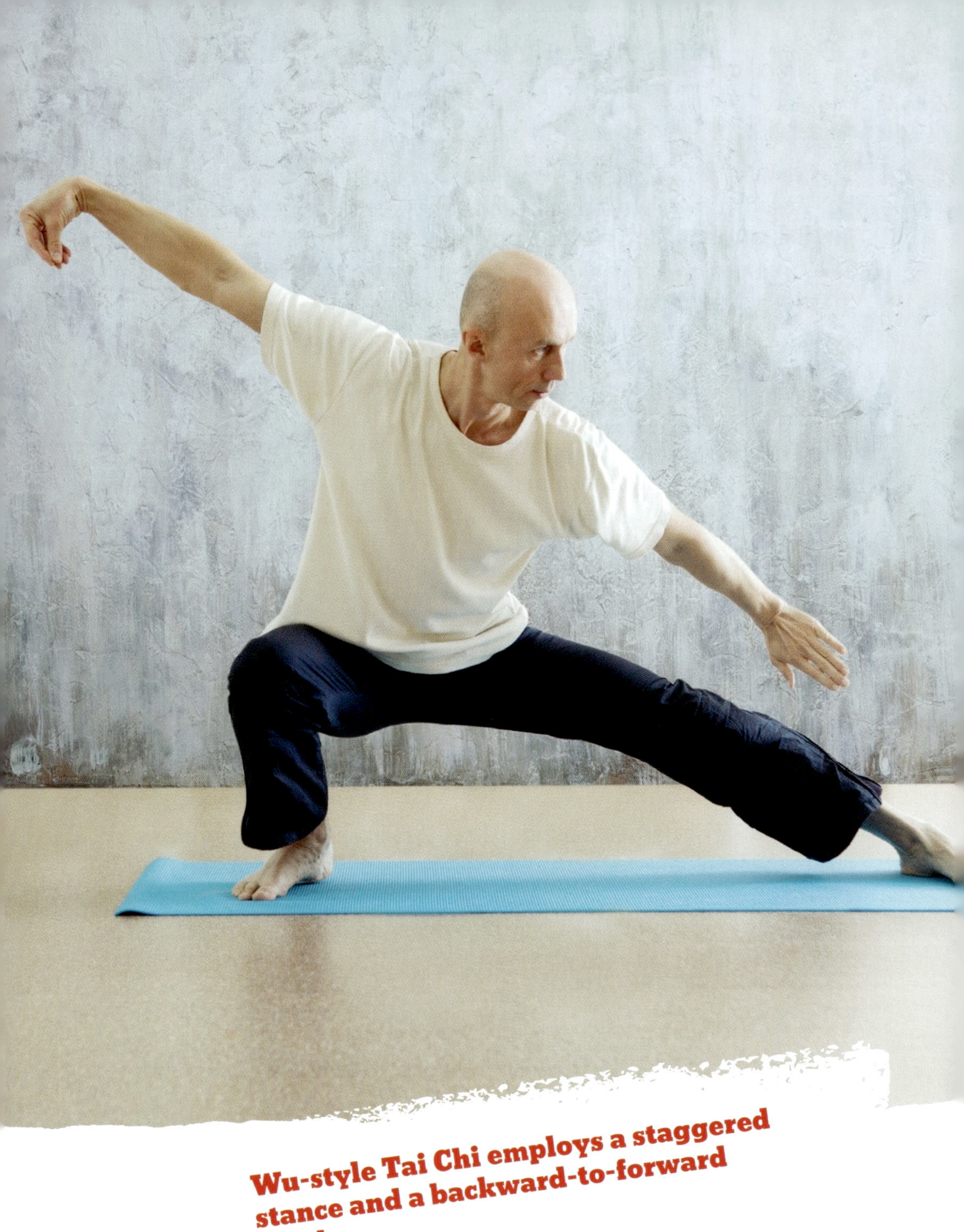

Wu-style Tai Chi employs a staggered stance and a backward-to-forward rhythm.

the body in a forward-to-backward rhythm. The back leg is staggered throughout this form of Tai Chi, which allows a sort of counterbalance that lets an individual fully extend their body without losing stability.

Sun Style

A Chinese scholar named Sun Lutang, already an expert in several other martial arts similar to Tai Chi, sought to implement a new form of the art that pulled together skills from the martial arts he was accustomed to, as well as existing versions of Tai Chi.

The Sun style places an emphasis on increasing agility. This is accomplished by incorporating a variety of leg and hip movements with the relaxed tempo present in most forms of Tai Chi. This technique combines fairly intricate footwork with flowing hand movements, forcing an individual to harmonize total-body movement patterns.

Hao Style

Widely regarded as the least popular style, the Hao variation of Tai Chi is also considered the most advanced. With this

FINDING WHICH STYLE OF TAI CHI IS BEST FOR YOU

Tai Chi can look quite a bit different depending on what variation is being practiced. When deciding what form is right for you, think about your own personal needs and weaknesses. If you are a more active individual looking to combine a strenuous workout with a mental edge, perhaps you are better suited for the Chen style. If you are a bit less mobile and simply want to improve your flexibility, the Yang style is probably your best bet. Whatever form of Tai Chi you adopt, you can be rest assured that there is a large body of research supporting this ancient art as a way to improve your physical and mental fitness.

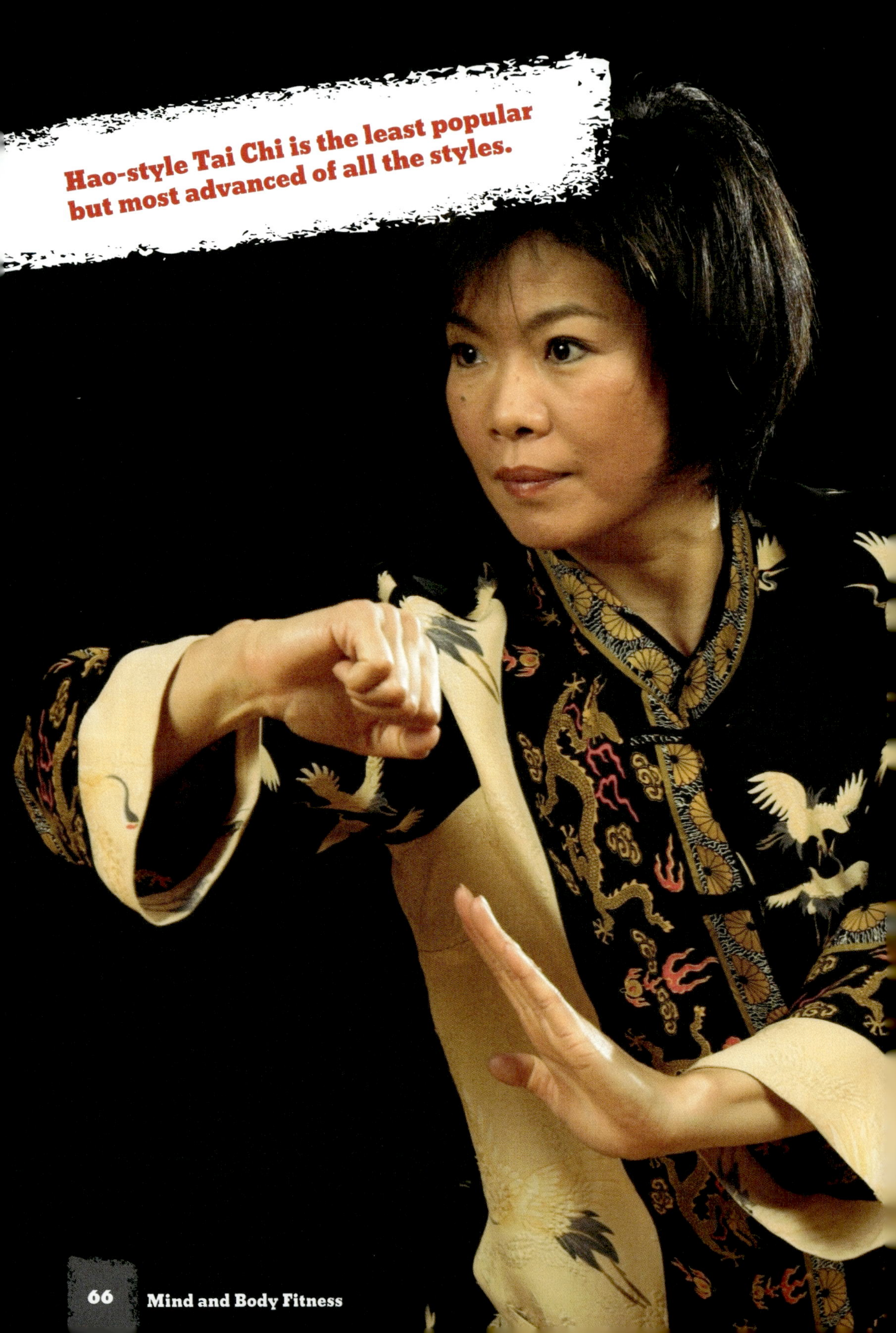

Hao-style Tai Chi is the least popular but most advanced of all the styles.

technique, there is a strong emphasis on enhancing internal energy (Qi). This involves performing what are described as strong internal movements to cause very small external movements. While performing the Hao style of Tai Chi, many of the movements seem to be very similar on the surface. This is due to the focus on channeling one's internal flow of energy.

TEXT-DEPENDENT QUESTIONS

1. What is the name of the individual most commonly credited with creating the earliest version of Tai Chi?
2. Of the five variations discussed, which form of Tai Chi most resembles a form of combat training?
3. What population of individuals might find more benefit in performing the Yang style of Tai Chi and why?

RESEARCH PROJECT

Chinese history is intricately related to the development of many forms of martial arts. While large portions of these styles are intended for self-defense, there is almost always a mental component included in each technique. Research another form of Chinese martial art that combines physical movement with mental focus. Describe in 250 words or less the origin of this technique and how it might be effective in improving your mind–body connection.

WORDS TO UNDERSTAND

catecholamine—any of various amines (such as epinephrine, norepinephrine, and dopamine) that function as hormones or neurotransmitters or both

excess post-exercise oxygen consumption (EPOC)—informally known as afterburn, this describes the theory that there is a physiological state after strenuous exercise in which the body continues to burn calories at an elevated rate for an extended period of time after the exercise has ended

neurotrophic—relating to or dependent on the influence of nerves on the nutrition of tissue

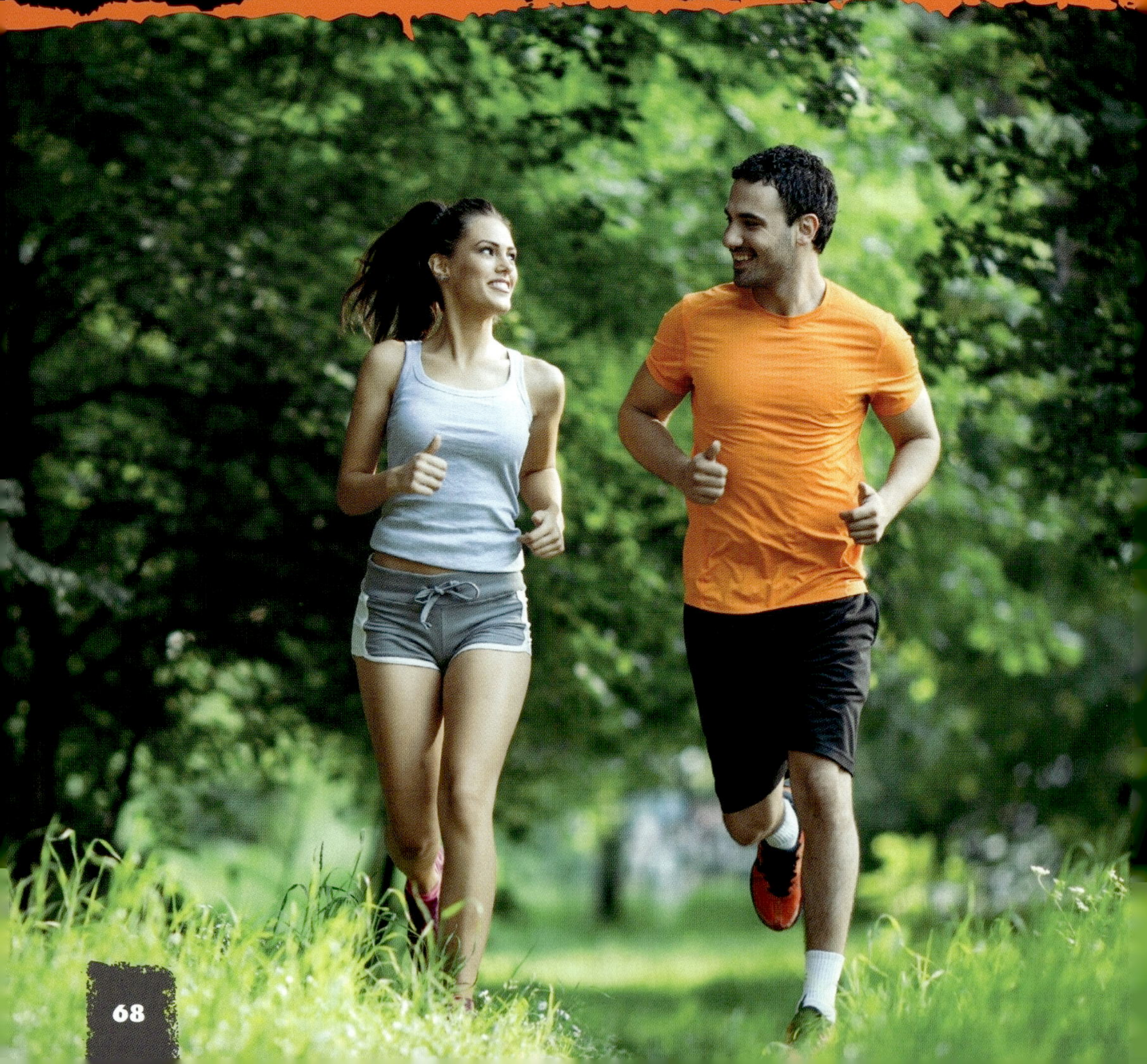

CHAPTER 6 RUNNING TOWARD A BETTER STATE OF MIND

The last method of working on your mental and physical fitness is a bit different than the rather elegant and sophisticated strategies discussed thus far. Even though you may consider running to be a purely physical endeavor, there is a large amount of research arguing the benefits of its use as a mental tool as well. As outlined in Chapter 3, exercise in general is beneficial to mental health. With that being said, any form of running, whether you prefer high-intensity sprints or a moderate-paced jog, will certainly benefit your body and mind in a big way.

RESEARCH SUPPORTING MENTAL BENEFITS OF RUNNING

Running brings to mind many different things for different individuals. For you, the word itself may signify a New Year's resolution you were fired up about that fell through the cracks. Maybe you are an athlete, meaning that the word run was usually yelled at your team by a coach as some punishment for a blunder at practice. Perhaps you are actually a huge fan of challenging yourself with a nice outdoor jog on a beautiful day.

Whatever the case may be, we will discuss some interesting research on the mental benefits of running. You are probably aware of some of the more commonly referred to benefits, such as the **catecholamine** rush usually known as the "runner's high." There are also many other reasons mental fitness can improve due to running.

This video briefly explains how running is an effective tool for building mind and body fitness.

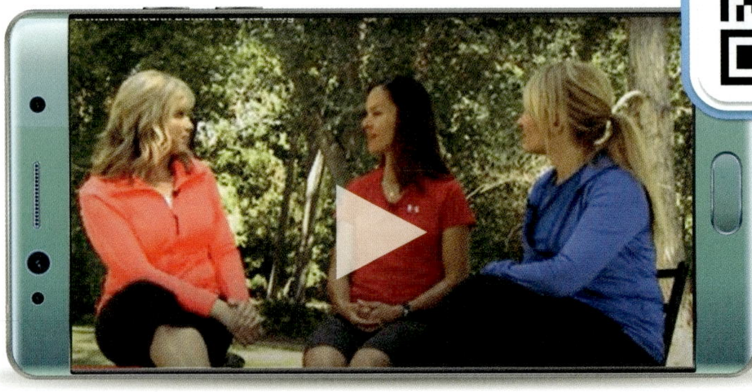

According to *Neurobiology of Learning and Memory,* running can actually improve your ability to learn! This journal describes a study in which researchers gathered a group of 27 participants, dividing them into two groups. One group began a running program, while the other did not perform any intervention at all. To assess any changes in learning ability, researchers tested each individual's ability to learn a new vocabulary. Further, several biological substances in the brain known to be associated with learning were measured, such as brain-derived **neurotrophic** factor (BDNF). At the conclusion of this experiment, the group of subjects that adhered to a running program improved their speed at which they learned the new vocabulary by 20 percent compared to the control group. Furthermore, the running group displayed significant increases in BDNF, whereas the control group did not.

Not only can running improve how well you learn, it can also slow down the aging process of your brain. *Time* magazine describes an interesting study published in the well-known neuroscience journal, *Neurology,* in which researchers wanted to find out if physical exercise or mental games were better at keeping the brain young. Six hundred and thirty-eight participants from Scotland were involved in this study, with each individual completing a survey at seventy years of age about their exercise routines, hobbies, and any mental activities or games

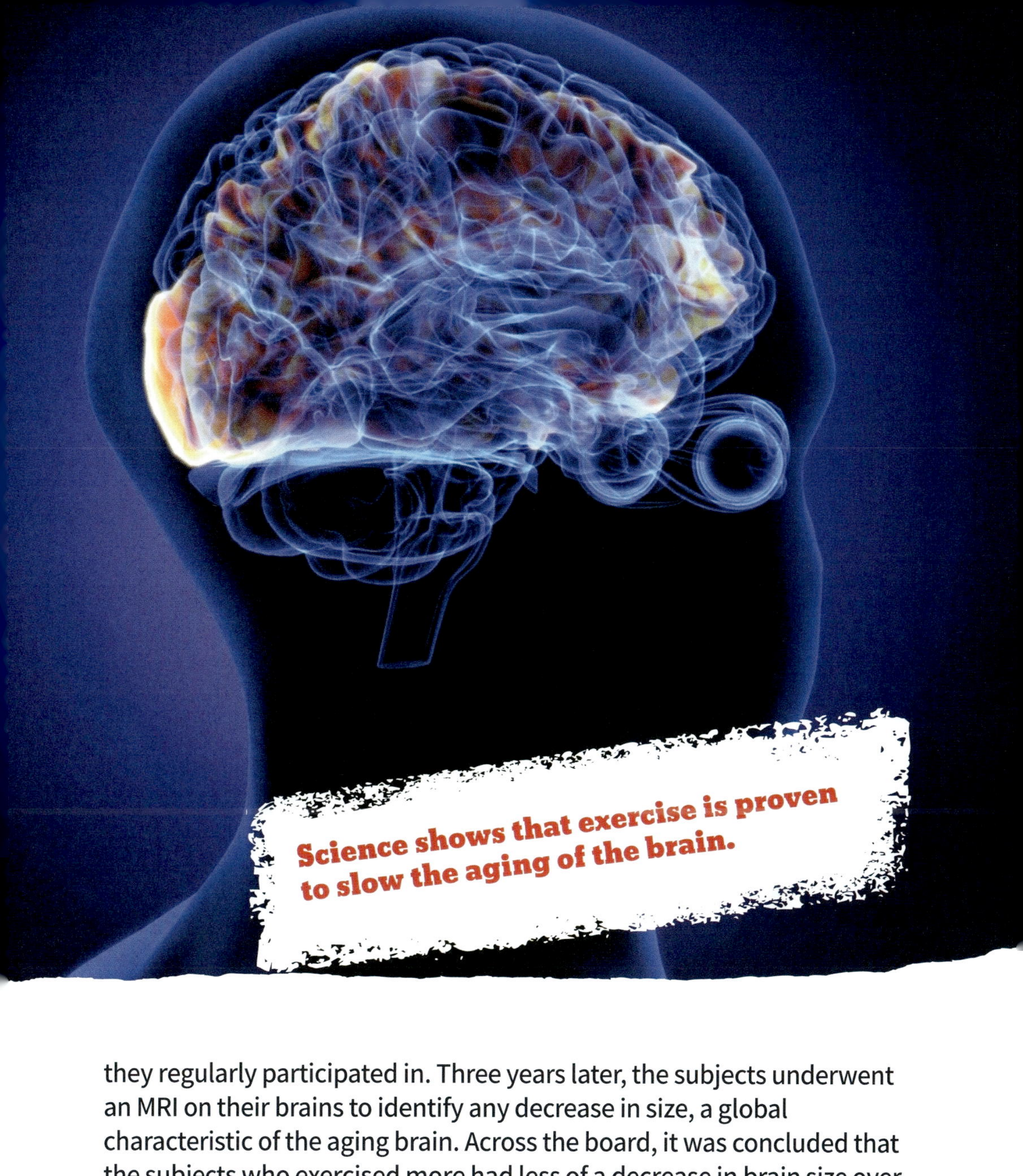

they regularly participated in. Three years later, the subjects underwent an MRI on their brains to identify any decrease in size, a global characteristic of the aging brain. Across the board, it was concluded that the subjects who exercised more had less of a decrease in brain size over the three-year period.

Unfortunately, a low sense of self-esteem is an issue many of us deal with today. More than ever before, we are tempted to compare ourselves with not only the people around us but people all over the world through outlets like social media. Although there are several effective ways to improve your self-esteem, running can actually be an asset. The *Journal of Adolescent Health* published a study that involved measuring the amount of physical activity (in the form of running) and self-esteem scores on 197 girls. Both these variables were assessed at ages nine, eleven, and thirteen. It was concluded that the more physical activity a subject performed, the higher her score on self-esteem inventories. Furthermore, more exercise at an earlier age was shown to be a reliable predictor of self-esteem at the next recorded age.

RUNNING IS FAR MORE THAN A PHYSICAL TASK

As human beings, our bodies are made to move. It is no surprise then that a generation of people more sedentary than ever before also possess the highest rate of mental health disorders. Running is something that comes naturally to humans; we do not prosper mentally or physically without exercise. If you need any more proof, consider this: human beings are the best endurance runners on the planet!

RESEARCH INTO THE PHYSICAL BENEFITS OF RUNNING

The way running improves physical fitness is by far the most obvious and well-known aspect of the activity. This is, in turn, good for your physical health, and there are few, if any, better arguments as to why you should do something than it making you live significantly longer. The research certainly shows that running may do just that. The *Journal of the American College of Cardiology* revealed that, in a study including more than 55,000 individuals, people who reported running as little as 5–10 minutes per day at very modest speeds

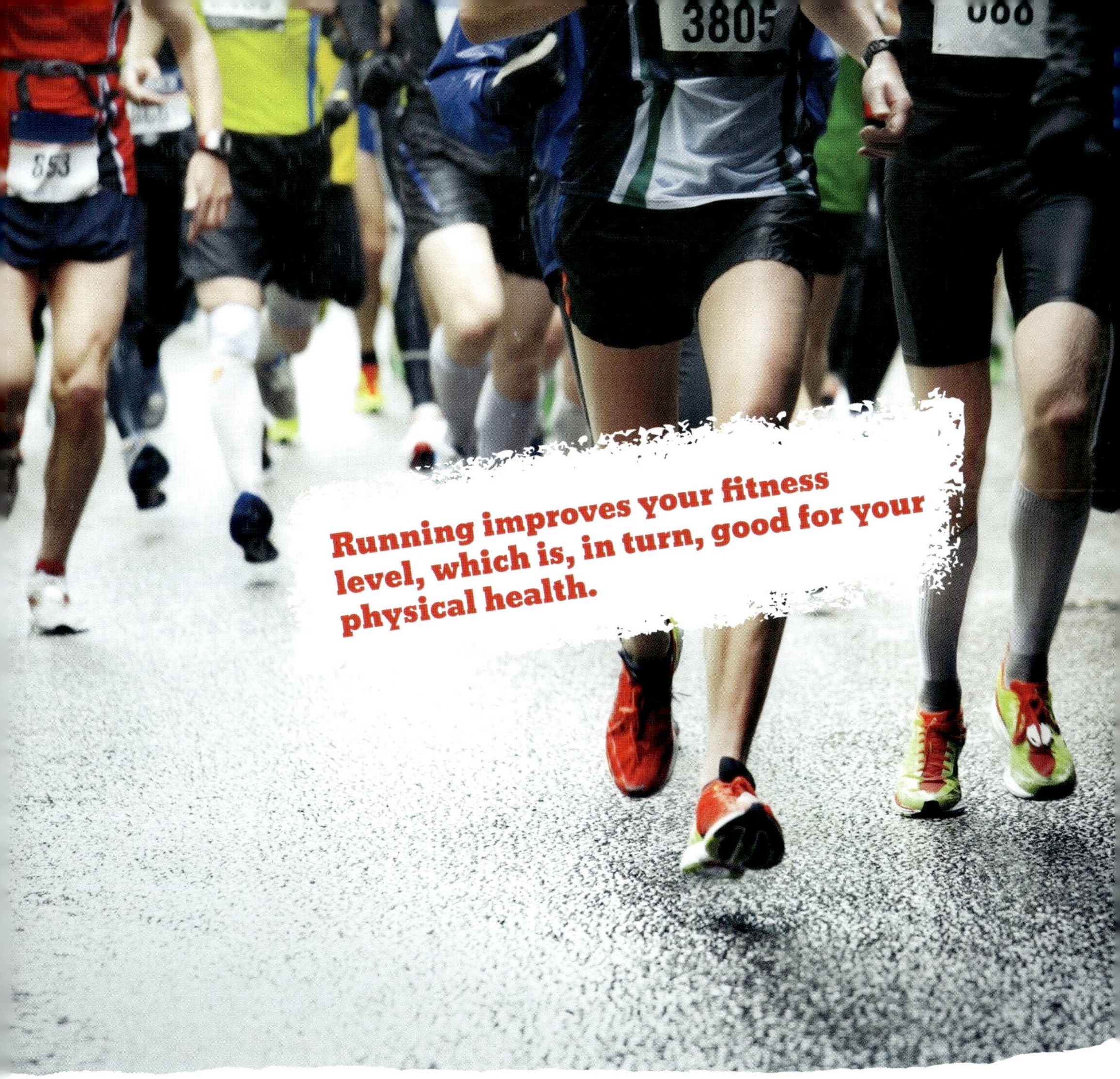
Running improves your fitness level, which is, in turn, good for your physical health.

(less than six miles per hour) lived an average of three years longer than their sedentary counterparts.

It is a pretty well-known fact that in order to lose weight, you need to burn more calories than you consume. It is also a fact that many people turn to walking and jogging as a way to accomplish this. However, a significant percentage of people say they consider walking and jogging pretty much the same in terms of effectiveness at cutting down on excess body fat. This is not the case. The research journal *Medicine and Science in Sports and Exercise* completed a study involving more

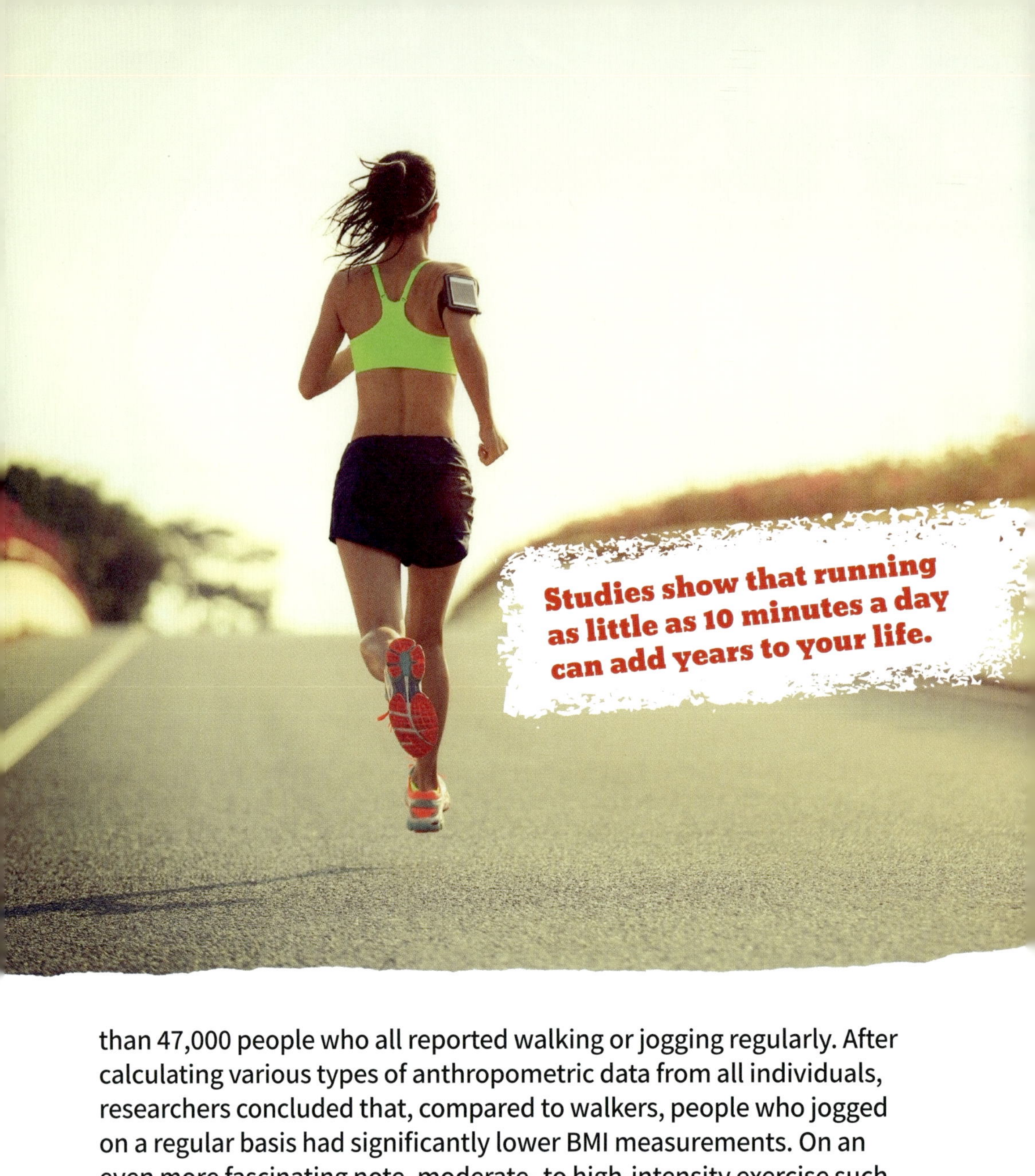
Studies show that running as little as 10 minutes a day can add years to your life.

than 47,000 people who all reported walking or jogging regularly. After calculating various types of anthropometric data from all individuals, researchers concluded that, compared to walkers, people who jogged on a regular basis had significantly lower BMI measurements. On an even more fascinating note, moderate- to high-intensity exercise such as running is associated with a theoretical process in your body, known as **excess post-exercise oxygen consumption** (EPOC). Put simply, the theory is that after you finish performing a strenuous physical activity, your body will actually keep burning calories at an elevated rate for quite a while, even after you are no longer exercising. The research to support this theory is inconclusive, however, but that would be quite a benefit if true.

The importance of maintaining a strong skeleton throughout every phase in life is a pretty obvious priority. When we are young, making sure our bones can handle the stress placed on them during intense sports and other physical activities prevents unnecessary injuries such as fractures. This becomes even more imperative as we age. Aging is associated with a significant decrease in skeletal mass and bone strength in men and women. Far too many older individuals lose their quality of life after a fall or accident in which they sustain a broken bone. Fortunately, the body is fascinatingly able to adapt to certain stimuli that encourage the formation of new bone tissue. Most of these stimuli are caused by repetitively putting stress on the bones in the form of resistance training or weight lifting. In regard to the legs, where the majority of skeletal injuries occur, running is a fantastic way to increase skeletal strength. A study published in the *American Journal of Public Health* looked at the relationship on 4,000 men. It was concluded that there was an almost perfect positive correlation between the amount of jogging the men reported and the strength of the largest bone in their legs.

MORE THAN A WEIGHT-LOSS TOOL

It is certainly true that aerobic exercise in any form, including running, is a viable way to burn calories and, thereby, helps people to lose weight. However, there are so many other physical benefits related to running for which it as rarely credited. If you have a bit, or even a lot, of excess weight you need to lose, taking up running is a good place to start. Doing this alone will improve your health in a big way. Just don't forget that besides improving any number on a scale, regular running benefits your body in so many other positive ways.

Running is proven to help increase the strength of leg bones.

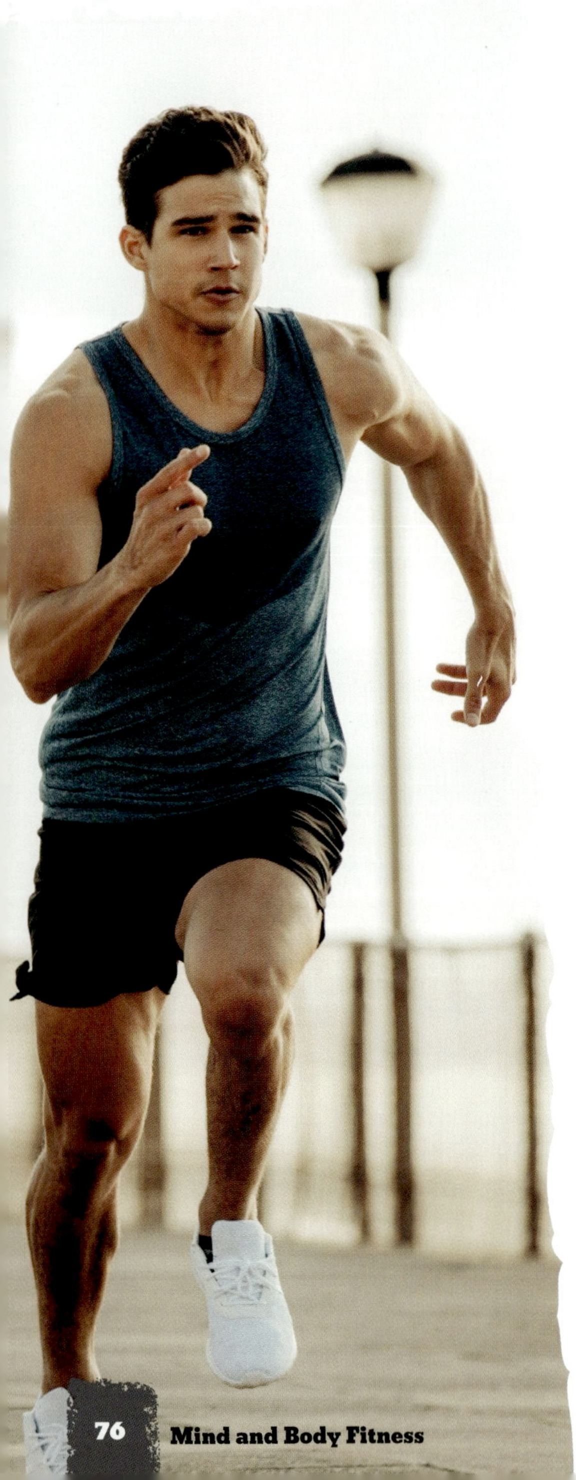

GETTING INTO RUNNING

If you find yourself in a place where even the thought of beginning a running program gives you nightmares of shin splints and pulled hamstrings, all is not lost. What you need to realize is that regardless of your current level of fitness, there is a way for you to begin to experience the mental and physical benefits of running in a manner that is sustainable and safe.

The key to getting started, as with every other form of exercise, is moderation. In no situation should you decide you want to begin running and immediately hit the pavement or track for hours on end. This is a sure-fire way to injure yourself and discourage you from continuing to try exercise programs. Instead, find a plan that allows you to begin running (or even walking) with even an extremely modest amount, progressing a little with each workout. There are plenty of free examples of these sort of

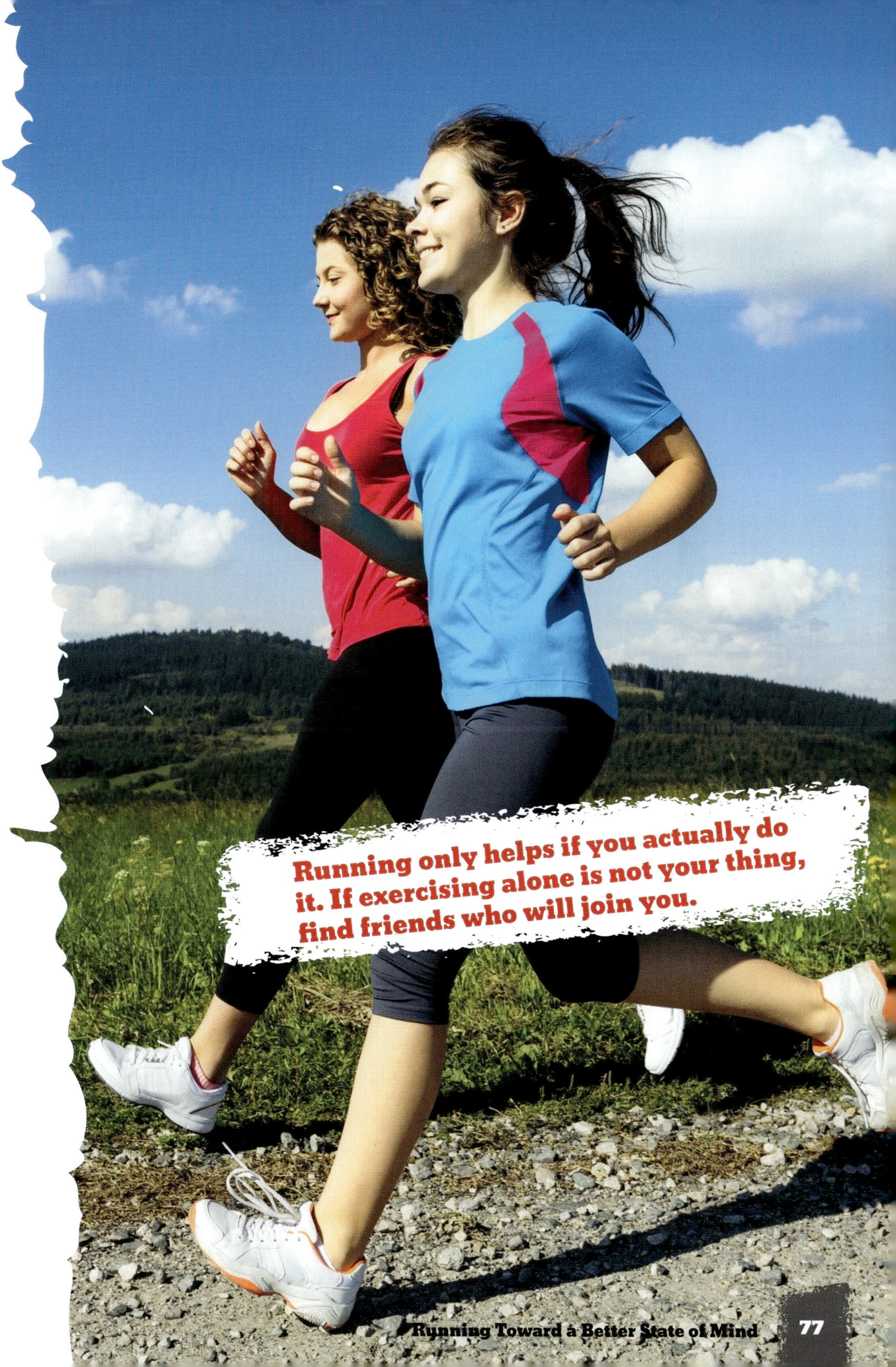

Running only helps if you actually do it. If exercising alone is not your thing, find friends who will join you.

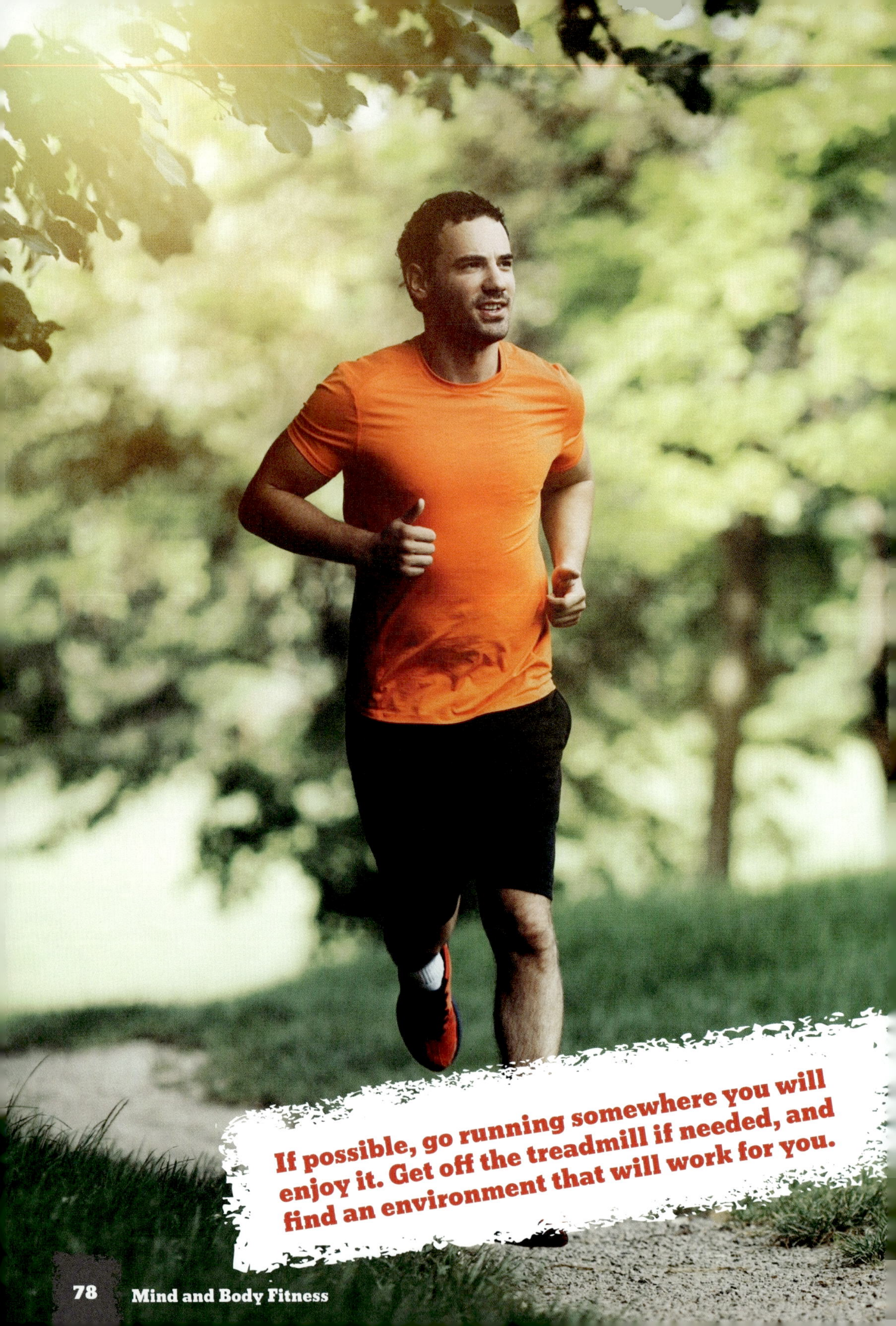

If possible, go running somewhere you will enjoy it. Get off the treadmill if needed, and find an environment that will work for you.

plans available online. Remember, you do not reap any of the benefits of running at a certain mileage; the results come from the challenge running imposes on your body. Think back to the study we talked about where researchers concluded that a slow jog even five minutes per day could help you live three years longer.

The level at which you start does not matter in the slightest. What is important is that you do start. If you are looking for a great way to improve your life in a multifaceted way, running might be your way to go.

TEXT-DEPENDENT QUESTIONS

1. According to the research mentioned in this chapter, what is the minimum amount of time an individual needs to run per day to extend their lifespan?
2. List two different mental health benefits mentioned in this chapter that have been linked to running according to the research.
3. How does running provide an effective way to strengthen the skeletal system?

RESEARCH PROJECT

In this chapter, we briefly touched on the EPOC effect that running has on your body. We discussed how you could continue to potentially burn calories even after you stop exercising. Dig a bit deeper into this effect and present arguments both for and against the existence of EPOC. Compile a chart presenting the opposing viewpoints and conclude which side seems more likely to be correct based on what you read. Be sure your sources base their opinions on credible science.

WORDS TO UNDERSTAND

homeostasis—a relatively stable state of equilibrium or a tendency toward such a state between the different but interdependent elements or groups of elements of an organism, population, or group

monotony—lack of variety and interest

vastus intermedius—the division of the quadriceps muscle that arises from and covers the front of the shaft of the femur

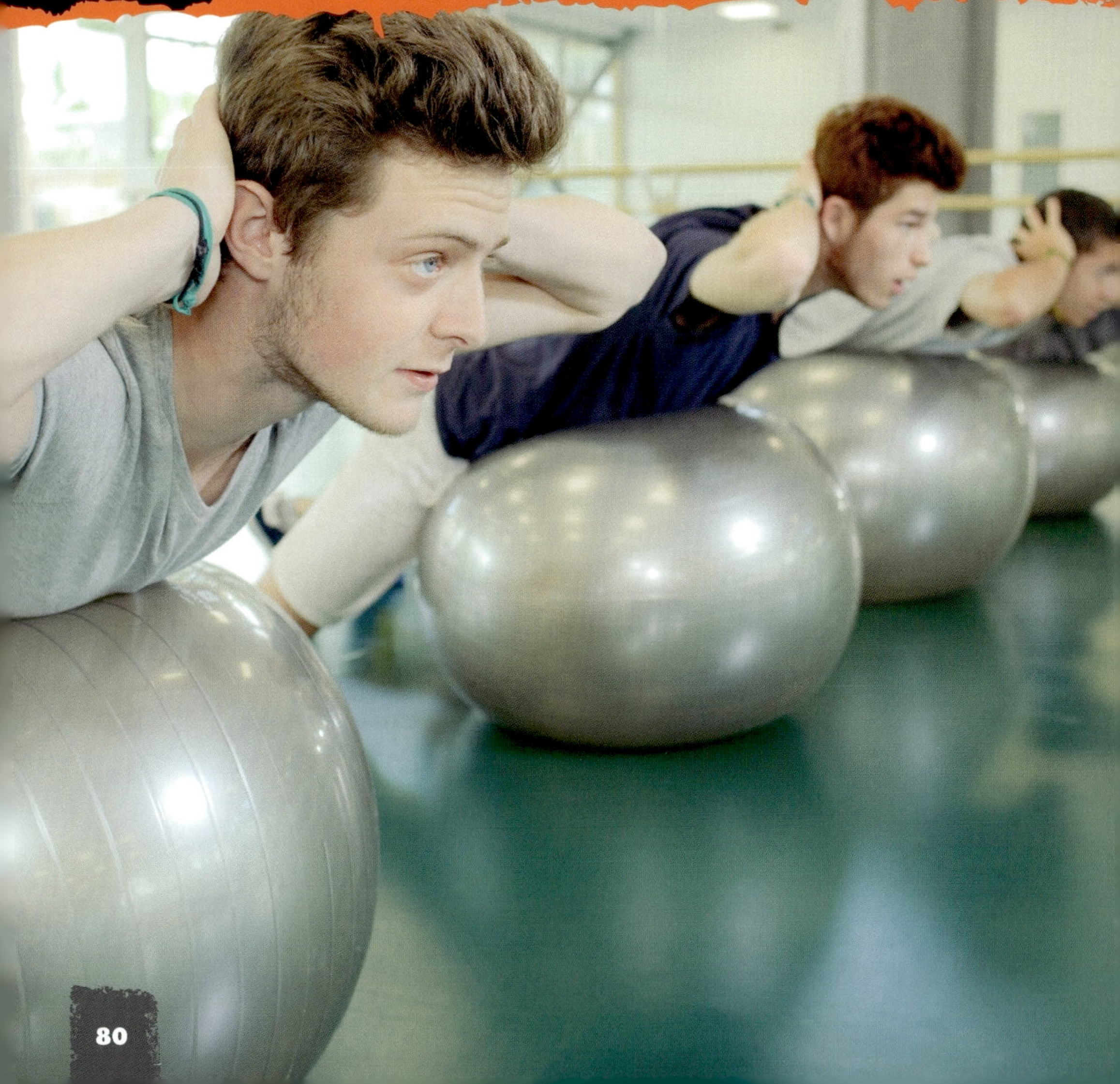

CHAPTER 7
DIVERSIFYING YOUR FITNESS ROUTINE

Keeping things new and exciting is an important aspect of fitness. This is an aspect of any self-improvement activity that often gets neglected. Working out and participating in a fitness program should be something that you look forward to doing. So much of our life is made up of things we don't really want to do, but that are required of us in one way or another. Due to this fact, adding anything else that you genuinely do not enjoy is only adding to the overall percentage of life spent on something other than being happy. A great aspect of fitness is that there are a multitude of ways to hone your mind and body, therefore providing plenty of options to find one you enjoy. Another way to promote happiness in regard to the way you exercise is diversity.

LIFE IS NOT MEANT TO BE STATIC (NEITHER IS FITNESS)

There are very few good things about **monotony**. Any way of life that involves repeating the exact same things day after day is usually not a fulfilling one. Since our time here may be short, we often aspire to fill it with new and exciting experiences. There are some things in life like school, work, and other responsibilities that seem to repeat themselves endlessly. Unfortunately, these are pretty much mandatory for most of us. What is important, then, is how you spend your time outside of the unavoidable commitments. The time that you do control is more enjoyable when filled with things that you are passionate about, things that excite you. Fitness is no different. The way you choose to improve your body and mind needs to be something you are happy to voluntarily do. The word voluntarily is important here, because exercise is a choice.

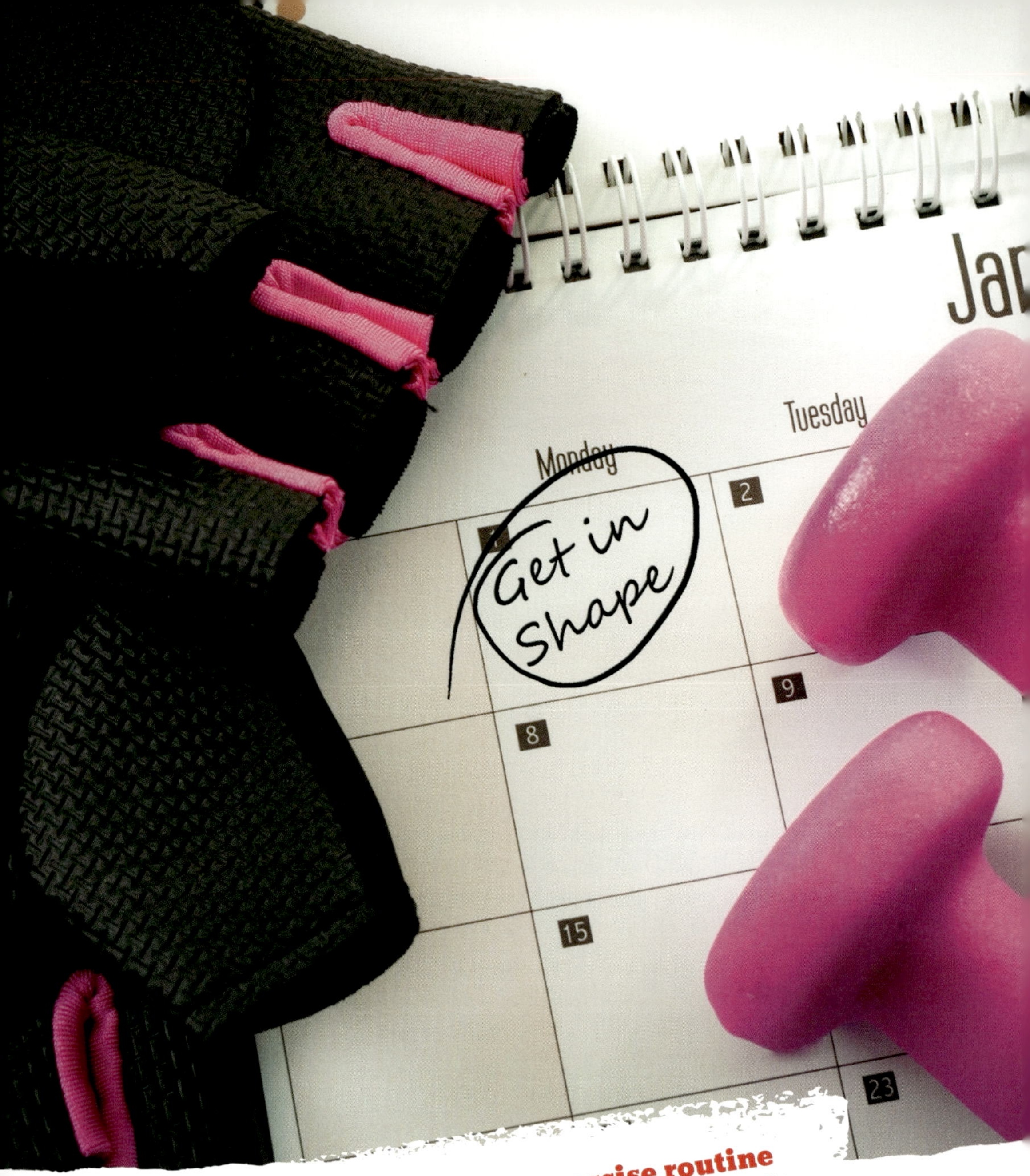

Getting started on an exercise routine is the first step, but it's sticking with it that brings the benefits.

Always be sure to try and diversify the way you work out in a way that it maintains its excitement.

WHY CHANGING YOUR EXERCISE METHOD IS GOOD FOR THE MIND

There is one key principle that is very helpful in obtaining the things you pursue in this life, and that is consistency. In fitness, for example, you can design the most effective workout program in the world, have an extremely dialed-in nutrition plan, and purchase the latest and greatest exercise gear out there, but if you are never consistently working out and eating right, your results will be limited, to say the least. How committed you are to fitness is far more important than the details of your plan. It is better to have a mediocre workout program in which you never miss a single day at the gym than to have an excellent plan where you only complete half your workouts.

One of the ways to remain consistent with your fitness routine is to enjoy what you are doing. This will require much less willpower. Human

EXERCISE IS NOT SUPPOSED TO BE PUNISHMENT

For one reason or another, many individuals are under the impression that exercise is some sort of necessary evil that we should all be subjected to. This is an unnecessarily negative outlook. While it is a fact that in order to experience an effective workout, you have to challenge your body, and that, yes, there is some discomfort involved, your perception is the difference maker. Instead of thinking about working out as some form of self-inflicted punishment, try to appreciate the opportunity you have to improve your body and mind on a routine basis.

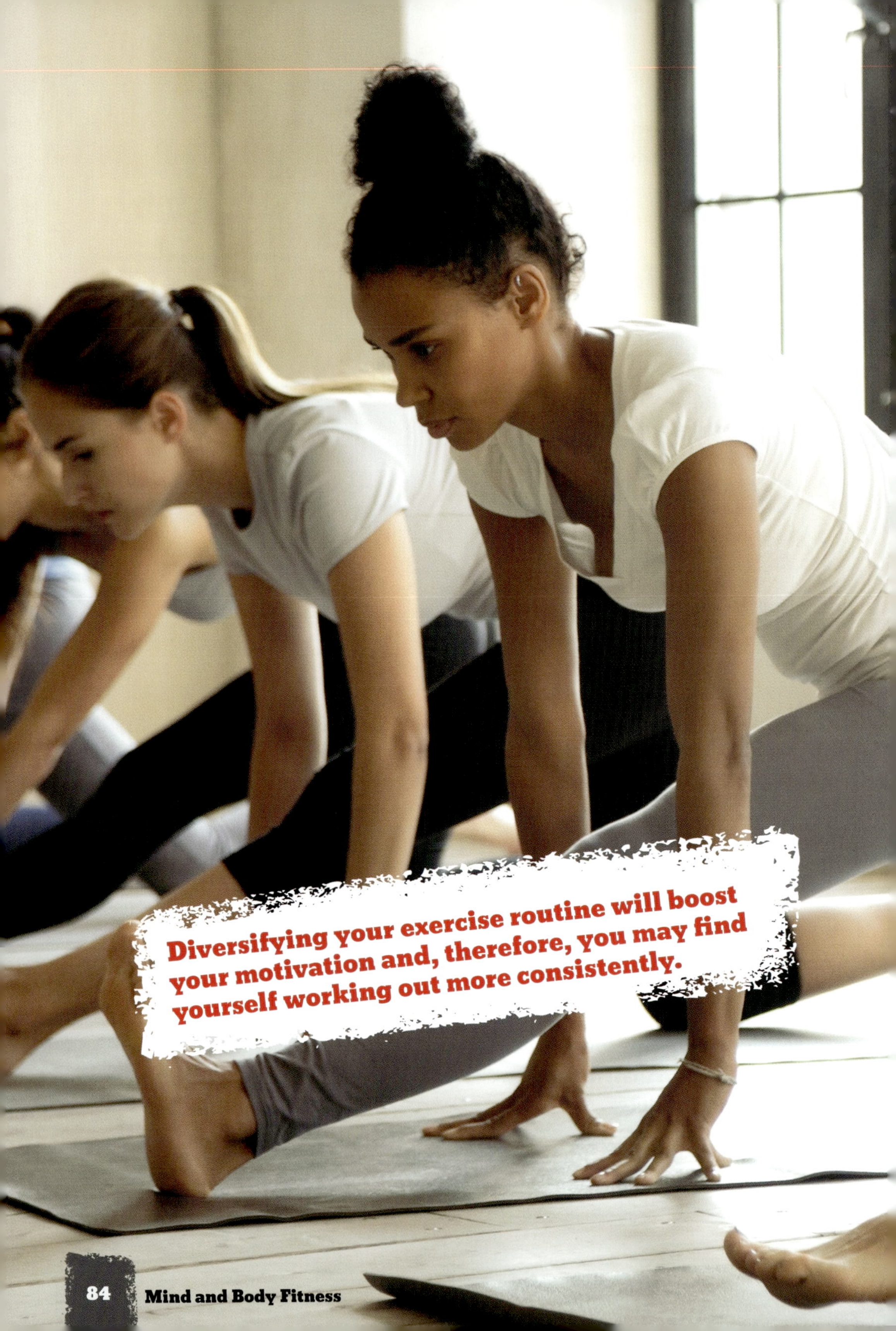

Diversifying your exercise routine will boost your motivation and, therefore, you may find yourself working out more consistently.

nature is extremely stubborn when it comes to avoiding things we dislike or that cause us a lot of discomfort. If you want to maximize your results, focus first on maximizing your consistency. Taking things one step further, it is important to discuss how to enjoy exercise. While there are a number of ways to accomplish this, diversifying the way you challenge your body is key. Even really enjoyable things become dull and boring if we experience them too often. Avoid being married to one workout method or ideology; don't let yourself fall into the routine of doing the exact same movements at the same place and time for months on end.

LIFE CONSTANTLY CHANGES, SO SHOULD YOUR WORKOUTS

If there is one certainty in life, it is that almost nothing is certain. From a practical standpoint, working out can be viewed simply as a way to prepare yourself to more effectively handle anything life throws your way. Therefore, it makes no sense to perform the exact same workout over and over. Start to think about your exercise routine as a carryover to your life in general. Change is inevitable; the way you challenge your body needs to reflect this.

There is, in fact, research supporting the idea that changing up your exercise selection is effective at boosting your motivation (and, therefore, consistency). The research journal *PLOS One* features an experiment in which researchers wished to determine whether working out using the same exercises or constantly changing exercises from workout to workout was better for increasing muscle thickness and boosting motivation. Twenty-one men were included in this experiment, and they were divided into two experimental groups according to both of the workout methods to be tested. At the end of eight weeks, both groups showed an increase in size of the quadriceps, the only difference being a slightly higher amount of growth of the **vastus intermedius** in the group doing the same exercises for each workout. However, the group that performed a large diversity of exercises during the eight-week period displayed a huge increase in their motivation versus their counterparts. When considering the importance of consistency in regard to fitness, a slight increase in the growth of a single muscle isn't nearly as important as the motivation to keep working out for the long run.

WHY CHANGING YOUR EXERCISE METHOD IS GOOD FOR THE BODY

Your body is extremely effective at making the necessary adaptations to continue functioning properly. This is the premise of **homeostasis**. When the body experiences a repeated stimulus for an extended period of time, it will change in some way to better respond to the stimulus. Something that is not discussed very often is the idea that homeostasis is the goal of working out and fitness in general. If you are consistently challenging your muscular system with weights, your body will see a need to adapt, and skeletal muscles will increase in size. Repeatedly performing a mindfulness exercise will result in your brain getting used to blocking out distractions and more effectively focusing your mental energy on the present moment.

While homeostasis is responsible for giving us the ability to change and improve our bodies, it is also the same biological response that requires us to keep changing the stimulus. If you continue to lift the same weight session after session, the muscle group you are using to lift the weight will of course grow and strengthen for a while. However, once the muscle has become strong enough to lift that weight without much effort, growth stops. At that point, it is necessary to either lift more weight or lift the same weight for more repetitions. The point is that for any improvement you hope to continue experiencing from a mental or physical perspective, diversity is the key. Your body is too good at adapting to its environment to continue changing unnecessarily.

Homeostasis

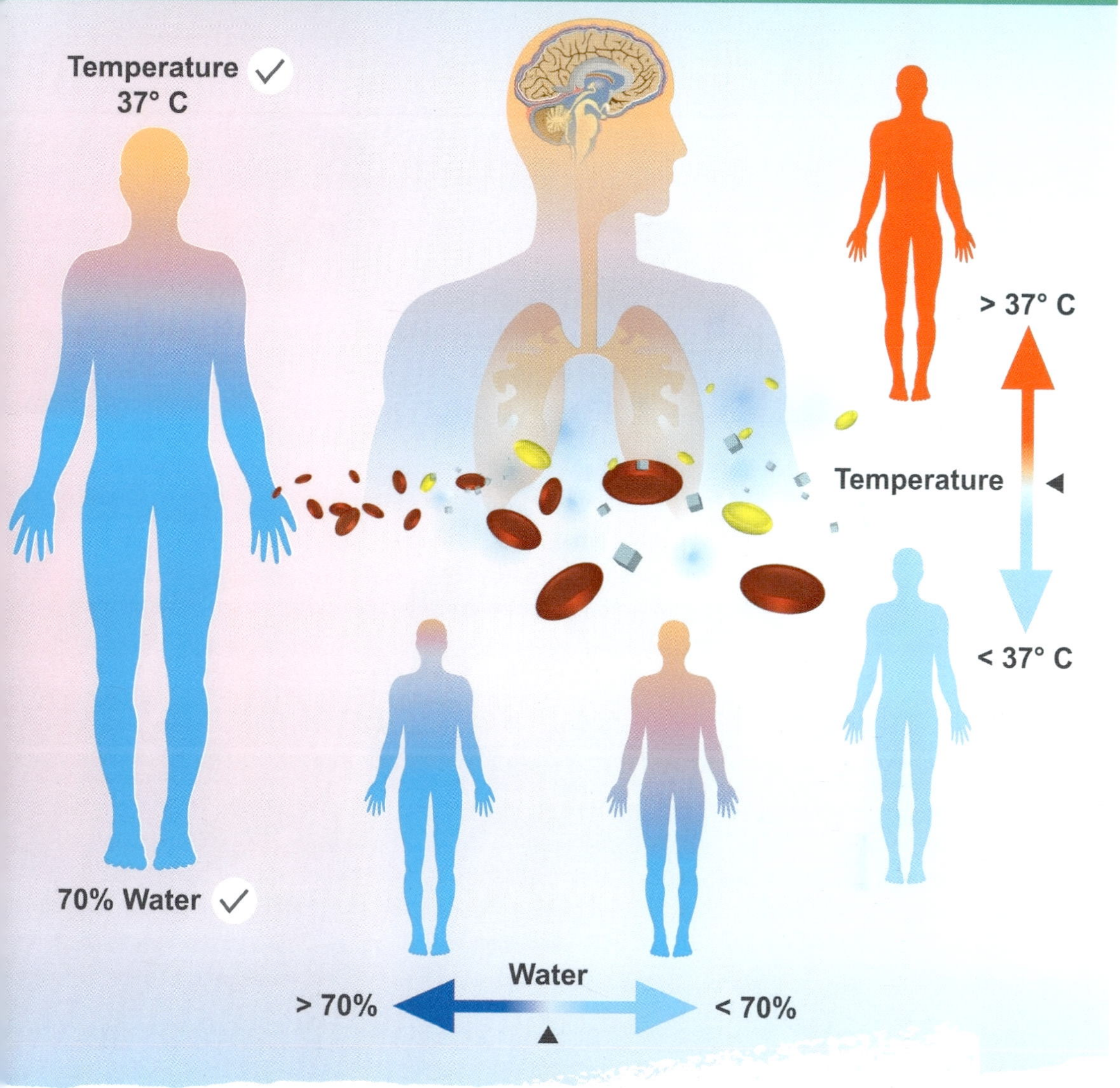

Homeostasis is where the body wants to be, so it will adapt to external stimuli until it gets there.

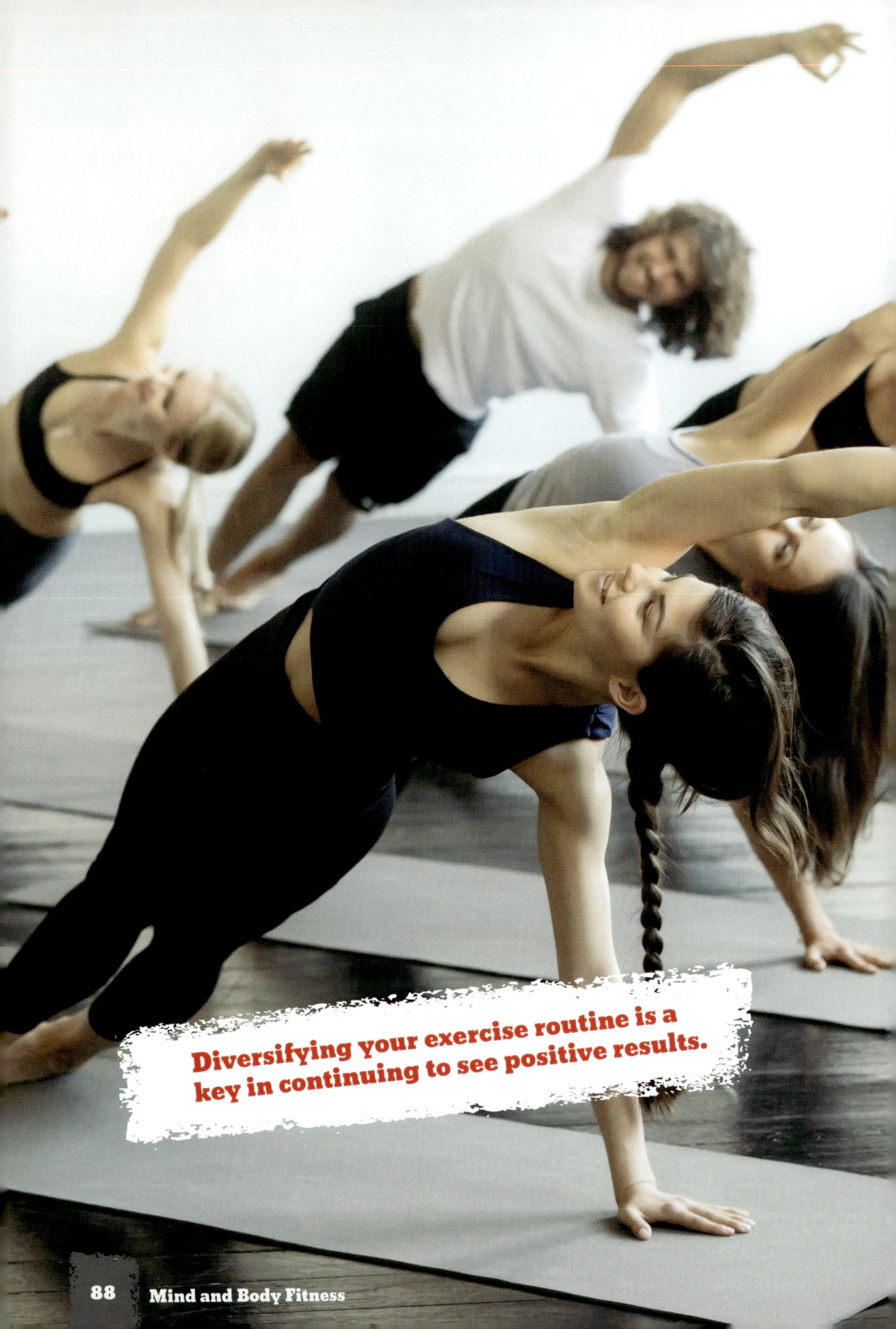

Diversifying your exercise routine is a key in continuing to see positive results.

Although the process of homeostasis is more-than-enough incentive to diversify your exercise routine, there is plenty of research available that reiterates this requirement. The *Journal of Strength and Conditioning Research* published a study in which 49 individuals were allocated into five different training groups. Each individual group was a diversified mix of people that focused on one of two different factors: intensity and exercise selection. Researchers chose to assess strength and muscle growth by recording the size of the quadriceps muscles as well as the one-rep maximum on the back squat for each individual before and after testing. After 12 weeks of adherence to their respected exercise routines, the group that worked out with the same intensity but varied their exercise selection over the course of the trial saw significant improvements over the other four groups. Not only did this group display significant growth in each of the four muscles that make up the quadriceps, they also increased the amount of weight they were able to perform on the back squat.

The evidence shows that changing up the way you exercise is important for the mind as well as the body. The human body is remarkable in its ability to adapt to changing circumstances in order to use as little resources as possible. If you want to see continued progress toward whatever your exercise goals may include (strength gain, muscle mass, weight loss), it is essential to continually give your body a reason to keep changing. Exercise variation can mean a lot of things such as changing the specific movement, engaging in a completely different form of training, even increasing the weight or repetitions used each workout. What is important is that you do it. Don't be afraid to get out of your normal routine and to challenge your body in a new way. Growth does not come from comfort.

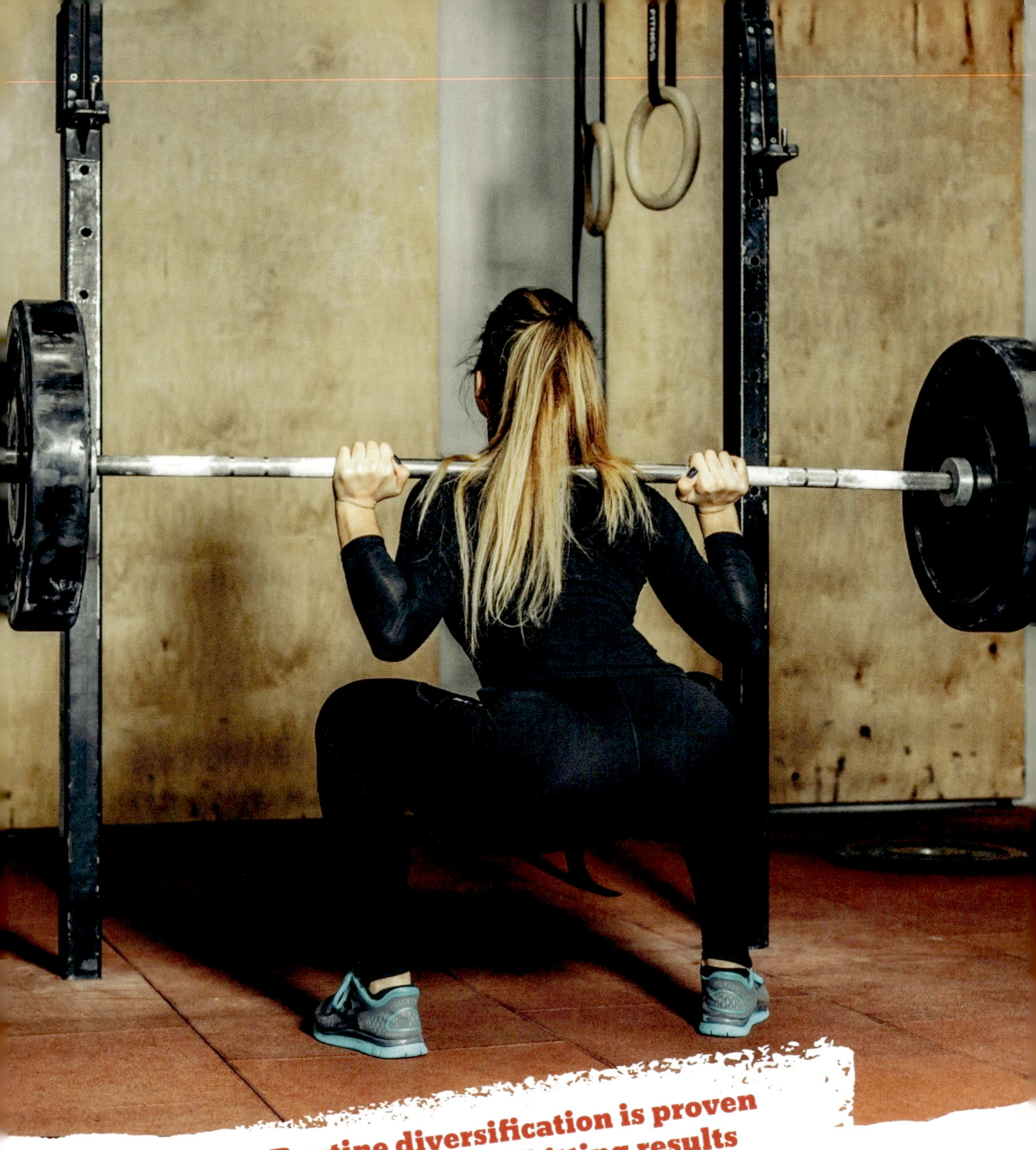

Routine diversification is proven not only to avoid hitting results plateaus but also to get superior results versus a uniform program.

This video does a good job of reiterating the physical benefits of switching up your workout routine.

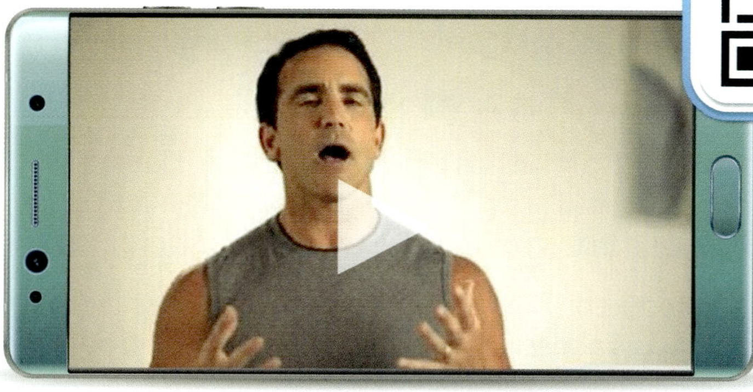

TEXT-DEPENDENT QUESTIONS

1. According to this chapter, what is the most important variable in seeing improvements in your fitness?
2. How does the concept of homeostasis apply to fitness in terms of making a continuous progress?
3. Why is it so important to make your fitness routine an enjoyable experience rather than something you dread having to do?

RESEARCH PROJECT

Think about all the different ways there are to improve your mental and physical fitness. Considering the importance of diversifying the way you exercise, do some research to help you design a one-week workout schedule. Using a week-long format, put together a plan that challenges you to utilize several different workout strategies that benefit you both physically and mentally.

SERIES GLOSSARY OF KEY TERMS

Cardiorespiratory – of or relating to the heart and the respiratory system.

Circuit training – a workout technique involving a series of exercises performed in rotation with minimal rest, often using different pieces of apparatus.

Fatigue – weariness or exhaustion from labor, exertion, or stress.

HDL cholesterol – also known as good cholesterol. A lipoprotein of blood plasma that is composed of a high proportion of protein with little triglyceride and cholesterol and that is correlated with reduced risk of atherosclerosis.

Hormone – a product of living cells that circulates in body fluids (such as blood) and produces a specific and often stimulatory effect on the activity of cells, usually remote from its point of origin.

Lactic acid – a normally present hygroscopic organic acid ($C_3H_6O_3$), especially in muscle tissue, that is a by-product of anaerobic glycolysis, produced in carbohydrate matter usually by bacterial fermentation, and used especially in food and medicine and in industry.

LDL cholesterol – also known as bad cholesterol. A lipoprotein of blood plasma that is composed of a moderate proportion of protein with little triglyceride and a high proportion of cholesterol and that is associated with increased probability of developing atherosclerosis.

Metabolism – the chemical changes in living cells by which energy is provided for vital processes and activities, and new material is assimilated.

Micronutrients – a chemical element or substance (such as calcium or vitamin C) that is essential in minute amounts to the growth and health of a living organism.

Modification – the making of a limited change in something, such as an exercise, that makes the exercise easier.

Physiology – a branch of biology that deals with the functions and activities of life or of living matter (such as organs, tissues, or cells) and of the physical and chemical phenomena involved.

Resistance – of, relating to, or being an exercise involving pushing or pulling against the source of an opposing force (such as a weight) to increase strength.

Tempo – rate of motion or activity.

FURTHER READING

Gunaratana, H. *Mindfulness in Plain English.* Somerville: Wisdom Publications, 2019.

Martin, C. *Yoga for Beginners: 35 Simple Yoga Poses to Calm Your Mind and Strengthen Your Body.* Berkeley: Rockridge Press, 2015.

Rilinger, H., and M. Murphy. *Lifted: 28 Days to Strengthen Your Body, Focus Your Mind, and Elevate Your Spirit.* Boston: Da Capo Life Long, 2017.

Rinpoche, S. M. *Running with the Mind of Meditation: Lessons for Training Body and Mind.* New York: Harmony, 2012.

INTERNET RESOURCES

www.experiencelife.com

This website is a great resource for providing information on improving your life both physically and mentally, the overall idea of this book.

www.mentalgamecoaching.com

Although this website also offers various certifications and products, there is an abundance of free content pertaining to mindfulness. This site also features information pertaining to the mental aspect of many different sports.

www.insanity-mind.com

This website is a fantastic collection of information and tips to improve a diverse array of mental components.

www.yogajournal.com

Yoga Journal is a user-friendly website that offers a ton of information related to various yoga techniques and instructional information on various poses.

www.runnersworld.com

This website provides advice and information related to virtually any aspect of running, from both a physical and mental perspective.

INDEX

AUTHOR BIOGRAPHY

Cole Johnson is a former college athlete, receiving numerous athletic honors related to athletic performance as well as excellence as a student-athlete. After graduating summa cum laude with a bachelor's degree in health science, he completed a doctorate of physical therapy program in 2020. As a lifetime health and fitness enthusiast with over five years of experience of producing fitness, exercise, and wellness content, he enjoys providing the audience with reliable, easy-to-understand information that readers can hopefully utilize to improve their overall quality of life.

PHOTO CREDITS

Shutterstock.com
Pg. 10: Flotsam, 11, 16, 18, 25, 49, 50, 52, 53, 54, 84, 88: fizkes, 13: PAUL ATKINSON, 14: VectorMine, 17: Phunkod, 21: mimagephotography, 22: Mikhailov Studio, 23: Antonio Guillem, 27: Yuganov Konstantin, 28: Sergey Nivens, 30: byswat, 32: Rost9, 34, 76: Jacob Lund, 35: Goran Bogicevic, 37: vmaslova, 38: siam.pukkato, 40: GP PIXSTOCK, 44: ittipon, 47: Helen Sushitskaya, 56: Juriah Mosin, 58: wavebreakmedia, 60, 61: May_Chanikran, 62: SBWorldphotography, 64: Ulza, 68, 78: nd3000, 71: Life science, 73: Mikael Damkier, 74: lzf, 77: Jacek Chabraszewski, 80: Phovoir, 82: Victor Moussa, 87: Studio BKK, 90: IvanRiver

Dreamstime.com
Pg. 1: Dmitry Molchanov, 3: Paultarasenko, 6: Motortion, 9: Nanci Mccraine, 42: Maryia Kazlouskaya

Wikimedia
Pg. 66: Keith Weng

EDUCATIONAL VIDEO LINKS

Chapter 1: http://x-qr.net/1LMw, http://x-qr.net/1M3e
Chapter 2: http://x-qr.net/1Hu3
Chapter 3: http://x-qr.net/1M3u, http://x-qr.net/1J9C
Chapter 4: http://x-qr.net/1L2z, http://x-qr.net/1M1y
Chapter 5: http://x-qr.net/1Lxa
Chapter 6: http://x-qr.net/1Ju6
Chapter 7: http://x-qr.net/1JST